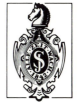

Peter Beighton · Rodney Grahame · Howard Bird

Hypermobility of Joints

With 101 Figures

Foreword by Professor Eric Bywaters

Springer-Verlag
Berlin Heidelberg New York 1983

Peter Beighton, MD, PhD, FRCP, DCH
Professor of Human Genetics and Director
MRC Research Unit for Inherited Skeletal Disorders
Medical School and Groot Schuur Hospital
University of Cape Town, South Africa

Rodney Grahame, MD, FRCP
Consultant Rheumatologist
Guy's Hospital, London, SE1 9RT, England

Howard Bird, MD, MRCP
Lecturer in Rheumatology, University of Leeds and
Consultant Rheumatologist, General Infirmary at Leeds
and Royal Bath Hospital, Harrogate, England

The cover of the book depicts a figurine of an Inca contortionist. It is reproduced by kind permission of the National Institute of Anthropology and History, Cordoba, Mexico.

ISBN 3-540-12113-7 Springer-Verlag Berlin Heidelberg New York
ISBN 0-387-12113-7 Springer-Verlag New York Heidelberg Berlin

Library of Congress Cataloging in Publication Data
Beighton, Peter. Hypermobility of Joints.
Bibliography: p. Includes index. 1. Joints — Hypermobility. I. Grahame, Rodney.
II. Bird, Howard, 1945– . III. Title. [DNLM: 1. Joint instability.
WE 300 B422h] RC933.B37 1983 616.7'2 83-347
ISBN 0-387-12113-7 (U.S.)

The use of general descriptive names, trade marks, etc. in this publication, even if the former are not to be taken as a sign names, as understood by the Trade Marks and Merchandise Marks Act, may accordingly be used freely by anyone.

Filmset by Polyglot Pte Ltd
Printed by William Clowes (Beccles) Limited, Beccles, Suffolk

2128/3916-543210

To our families, to Lax Lizzie (who started it all),
and to our hypermobile patients everywhere.

Foreword

Although those of us (and particularly orthopaedists and rheumatologists) who deal with locomotor diseases in man are concerned mainly with stiffness and limitation of movement— affecting not only livelihood but also the quality of life—from time to time we see patients suffering from too much of a good thing, whose joints are too freely mobile for the good of the whole man. In most instances, at least in youth, the benefit outweighs the debit. Many hypermobile people in the performing world— ballet dancers, circus gymnasts, musicians and sportsmen and women—have delighted audiences over 20 centuries with their unusual ability, prowess and postures. Some types of acquired hypermobility can, however, be disadvantageous, an example being tabes dorsalis with its flaccid joints and perhaps pain as well.

In a similar way the restored-to-normal mobility of treated rheumatoid patients (whether by prednisone or longer term drugs such as penicillamine or gold) must be considered abnormal—as hypermobility for that patient which in the long-term may hasten secondary arthrotic changes.

This treatise deals, however, with the abnormally mobile, either as an effect of inherited connective tissue abnormality or as one end of the normal range of mobility, without any obvious connective tissue change. It comes at a fecund time in our knowledge of the intricacies of the collagen molecule, with intriguing questions concerning the development of local type-specific structures. The fibroblast may yet expand to the same diversity as the once humble lymphocyte.

I first encountered this generalised "hypermobility syndrome" in a young doctor in 1950 (Kirk et al. 1967) and by the 1960s the syndrome (for that is all it is) had become well known. These patients had often been passed from doctor to doctor, from one consultant to another, with no relief, no understanding and no diagnosis other than "fibrositis" or its more modern 1960s equivalent, "psychogenic rheumatism". Although there was nothing that could pass as a cure, we found that explanation to the patient of the nature of his pains was of very considerable value and in itself therapeutic.

The authors of this book have each contributed in large measure to our modern knowledge of this field; here the various aspects of hypermobility (or hyperlaxity) are brought together for the first time, covering a surprisingly wide field: not only heritable diseases involving collagen assembly (whose present position is well stated) and elastin (about which much less is known) but also genetic, developmental, social, occupational, cardiovascular and locomotor aspects, even if we know little about them as yet. Fields for further exploration abound. Ethnic differences are very obvious but few population comparisons have been made: the literature is full of unascertained guess-work ("Perhaps hence the apparent pre-eminence of Egyptians in belly-dancing". Bywaters 1981). No mention is made of animal models—perhaps not yet observed, but a powerful help in other fields. There is still opportunity for further prospective clinical research in regard to the long-term course and complications of this anomaly. Finally, since hypermobility is common with us and commoner still in other races, we need to know what effect it has on the course and severity of other locomotor diseases, such as RA, other cardiovascular problems, such as mitral valve prolapse, and (still unexplored) eye-ball and tooth changes needing inter- and intraracial comparisons.

I congratulate the authors for providing an up-to-date platform to encourage further exploration of a potentially rich field.

References

Kirk JH, Ansell BM, Bywaters EGL (1967) The hypermobility syndrome. Ann Rheum Dis 26: 419–425
Bywaters EGL (1982) Mobility with rigidity: a view of the spine. Ann Rheum Dis 41: 910–214

January, 1983   Professor E. G. L. Bywaters
CBE, FRCP, FACP, FRCP (Canada)
Emeritus Professor of Rheumatology
Royal Postgraduate Medical School
of London

Preface

Persons with an excessive range of joint movements are regarded as being 'hypermobile' and it is becoming increasingly apparent that joint laxity is of considerable importance in clinical practice. Our purpose in writing this book is to combine our longstanding interests in different facets of hypermobility in an up-to-date review of the subject as a whole.

It has been argued that the word 'hypermobility' is inaccurate in its medical context and that it should be replaced by 'hyperlaxity' or 'hyperextensibility'. However, for the sake of clarity we have adhered to the terminology used in previous publications and we have employed these terms interchangeably.

Semantic and nosological problems also exist concerning the designation 'hypermobility syndrome'. In rheumatological practice the term is applied in a general sense to any loose jointed patient with musculo-skeletal symptoms. A small proportion of these persons have well-defined genetic disorders, but in the majority no specific syndromic diagnosis can be made. There is controversy as to whether these individuals represent the upper end of the normal spectrum of articular movements, or whether they have a distinct, but poorly differentiated, collagen disorder. This problem is discussed at appropriate points in the text.

We have described the existing clinical and biometrical methods for assessment of the range of joint movements in individuals and populations, and have discussed the practical application of these techniques. The pathogenesis of hypermobility is bound up with the structure and function of connective tissue and we have therefore given a simple outline of the relevant histopathology, collagen chemistry and biomechanics.

Hypermobility is important in rheumatological practice because excessive joint laxity produces a wide variety of articular complications. Hypermobility also has special implications for many fields of activity, including sport and the performing arts. In the genetic context joint laxity is a component of numerous heritable syndromes. Although individually rare, these disorders are collectively not uncommon and they are reviewed in the final chapters.

We have written this book because we believe that the time is ripe for the existing knowledge concerning articular hypermobility to be presented in a comprehensive manner. We hope that our work will be of interest to rheumatologists and orthopaedic surgeons, but loosely speaking, this book contains information for internists and colleagues in many other disciplines, including medical genetics, paediatrics, physiotherapy, collagen chemistry and bioengineering.

January 1983   Peter Beighton
                                                Rodney Grahame
                                                Howard Bird

Acknowledgements

We wish to thank all those who have provided assistance:

RA de Méneaud for preparing the illustrations;

June Chambers for typing the manuscript;

Dr J Cornell and Mr F Horan for their critical appraisal of the manuscript;

Colleagues who have facilitated or been directly involved in our investigations, notably Professor George Dall, Louis Solomon, Verna Wright, Wilson Harvey and Anne Child;

Many physicians who, over the years and knowing of our interest, have referred patients with hypermobility of joints;

The Arthritis and Rheumatism Council for Research in Great Britain and the Commonwealth, the Medical Research Council of South Africa and the University of Cape Town Staff Research Fund for financial support for investigations related to hypermobility;

Michael Jackson of Springer-Verlag for his benign tolerance and good-humoured encouragement.

Contents

Section I
Basic Aspects of Hypermobility

1. Introduction to Hypermobility

Historical Background

The first clinical description of articular hypermobility is attributed to Hippocrates who, in the fourth century B.C., described the Scythians, a race of people inhabiting the region that now forms the Ukraine and Czechoslovakia, as having humidity, flabbiness and atony such that they were unable to use their weapons. Their main problem in warfare was that hyperlaxity of the elbow and shoulder joints prevented them from effectively drawing their bows.

Thereafter the study of joint hypermobility was ignored until the late nineteenth century when general physicians were energetically defining medical syndromes, some of which included joint hypermobility as an important feature. Notable amongst these were the Ehlers–Danlos (EDS) and the Marfan syndromes.

The last 50 years have seen the recognition of joint hypermobility, without more widespread connective tissue abnormality, as a cause of orthopaedic and rheumatological symptoms. In investigations on a small number of subjects Finkelstein (1916) and Key (1927) noted a familial predisposition to lax joints. Subsequently orthopaedic surgeons recognised the importance of generalised joint laxity in the pathogenesis of dislocation of a single joint. Congenital dislocation of the hip was investigated by Massie and Howarth (1951) and Carter and Wilkinson (1964). Carter and Sweetnam studied dislocation of the patella (1958) and dislocation of the patella and shoulder (1960). Thereafter generalised joint laxity was recognised as being more common than had previously been realised. This led to the introduction of simple clinical scoring systems for measuring joint laxity in affected individuals and populations.

The first report of an association between joint laxity and rheumatological symptoms emanated from Sutro (1947) who described 13 young adults with effusions and pain in hypermobile knees and ankles. Similar clinical observations led Kirk et al. (1967) to define the 'hypermobility syndrome' in a group of patients with joint laxity and musculoskeletal complaints. In the absence of demonstrable systemic rheumatological disease, these authors attributed the symptoms to articular hypermobility.

Wood (1971) argued from the epidemiological viewpoint that joint hyper-mobility should be considered as a graded trait rather than as an 'all or nothing' syndrome. This is a simplistic concept, and there is general agree-ment amongst colleagues with clinical experience that the category of loose-jointed persons contains not only those at the upper end of the normal spectrum, but also examples of familial undifferentiated hypermobility syndromes (see Chap. 10).

Development of Concepts Concerning Rheumatological Manifestations

It is apparent that symptoms arising from lax joints may commence at any age. In their classical paper, Kirk et al. (1967) described 24 patients with generalised joint hypermobility. Their symptoms started between the ages of 3 and 55, and three-quarters had problems before the age of 15. Females were more frequently affected than males. Symptoms were mainly in the lower limbs, the commonest being pain in the knees and ankles, although joint effusions and muscle cramps also occurred. Supraspinatus and bicipital tendonitis, tennis elbow and painful Achilles tendons were also noted.

In a comprehensive review Ansell (1972) mentioned that symptoms occur after, rather than during, unaccustomed exercise and diminish in later life, perhaps as the joints stiffen. Although the prognosis is good, other arthro-pathies must be excluded before making a diagnosis of the 'hypermobility syndrome'. Thus, in 690 new referrals to a paediatric rheumatology unit, hypermobility was considered to be the final diagnosis in only 12. Most clinicians agree that the condition is under-diagnosed, and with greater awareness many patients with 'growing pains' in childhood are likely to be recognised as hypermobile.

Some persons consider themselves to be 'double-jointed' or 'loose-limbed'. There is often a family history of loose joints, and they may be talented at activities such as ballet dancing (see Chap. 8). By contrast, symptomatic patients are sometimes labelled as neurotic when medical practitioners, who are unaware of the syndrome, are unable to explain their symptoms.

The hypermobile individual may be especially at risk from chronic back pain, disc prolapse and spondylolisthesis. In addition the 'loose back' syndrome, in which women with hypermobility develop unexplained back pain in the absence of demonstrable disc lesions or spondylitis, is now accepted as being more common than originally supposed (Howes and Isdale 1971).

Extra-articular Manifestations of Hypermobility

There is a paucity of studies on the extra-articular manifestations of familial hypermobility. However, the collagen present in the joint capsules and ligaments is found elsewhere in the body, and it would be surprising if joint hyperlaxity was not a component of a generalised systemic disorder in some persons. There is a strong impression that individuals with loose joints are susceptible to varicose veins, herniae and rupture of lung tissue leading to pneumothorax. In addition, it is becoming increasingly evident that mitral valve prolapse (floppy mitral valve syndrome) is associated with articular hypermobility (see Chap. 5).

Dermal hyperelasticity is sometimes present in individuals with hypermobile joints and various methods for measuring the physical properties of skin have been devised. These techniques have been used in EDS (Grahame and Beighton 1969) and in population studies (Grahame 1970, Silverman et al. 1975).

Late Effects of Hypermobility

Throughout the literature it is widely held that premature osteoarthrosis may be a direct consequence of hypermobility. However, final proof may only come from a large and prospective long-term study with adequate controls. In an investigation of EDS, which exhibits classical hypermobility, 16 out of a group of 22 individuals over the age of 40 had clinical osteoarthrosis. The six persons without osteoarthrosis had significantly less joint laxity (Beighton et al. 1969). Premature osteoarthrosis was a feature of the hypermobile patients in the original studies of Kirk et al. (1967); all affected patients were female with an age of onset of symptoms of 33–56 years. The trapezio-metacarpal joints and the cervical spine were the commonest sites of involvement in this group.

In a radiological, histological and arthroscopic study Bird et al. (1978) drew attention to the way in which joint hyperlaxity apparently predisposes to a traumatic synovitis in the third decade and premature osteoarthrosis in the fourth or fifth. Pyrophosphate is subsequently deposited in the unstable joint.

The articular complications of hypermobility are reviewed in detail in Chap. 5.

Measurement of Joint Hypermobility

Clinicians and epidemiologists agree on the need to measure joint laxity. The first scoring system was devised by Carter and Wilkinson (1964) and subsequently modified by successive authors (Grahame and Jenkins 1972; Horan and Beighton 1973). The method which has gained general acceptance is that derived by Beighton et al. (1973) from the earlier scheme of Carter and Wilkinson. In this technique a score of 0–9 is allocated to each individual, the highest scores denoting maximum joint laxity. Although more complex systems have been proposed, they are time consuming and have not been widely used.

There is a substantial body of literature concerning the measurement of movements at individual joints. Methods include radiological assessment (Harris and Joseph 1949), photographic techniques (Troup et al. 1968) and the pendulum machine devised by Barnett (1971) for the calculation of the coefficient of resistance in the interphalangeal joints.

Complicated or invasive techniques cannot be used in large population studies and there has been a swing back to simple methods. Grahame and Jenkins (1972) constructed a device to measure the angle of extension at the little finger when a standard force is applied. To some extent this has been superseded by the Leeds Finger Hyperextensometer, which records the range of movement at the metacarpophalangeal joint of the index finger in response to a pre-set torque. Methods of assessment of joint mobility are reviewed in detail in Chap. 2.

Syndromic Associations of Joint Hypermobility

Although no demonstrable hereditary disorder of connective tissue can be recognised in the majority of individuals with joint hypermobility, a proportion have specific genetic conditions such as EDS, familial undifferentiated hypermobility and the Larsen syndromes (see Chaps. 9, 10 and 11).

It is sometimes extremely difficult to diagnose minor forms of disorders of connective tissue. The characteristic picture of the complete Marfan syndrome with long thin limbs, ectopia lentis and dilatation of the ascending aorta is easily recognised, but a definitive diagnosis is difficult in persons with mild manifestations. Separation is even more difficult in the case of the 'Marfanoid Hypermobility Syndrome' (Walker et al. 1969), which lacks eye and aorta involvement yet is characterised by gross joint laxity and hyperelastic skin. Similarly, although some varieties of EDS are easy to recognise, the benign hypermobile type III can closely mimic the familial undifferentiated hypermobility syndrome in both clinical presentation and mode of inheritance (Beighton et al. 1969).

Finally, it is of practical importance that joint hypermobility can occur as a secondary manifestation of inflammatory disorders such as rheumatoid arthritis. In these circumstances the clinical picture is sometimes complicated by the presence of a neuropathy which may accentuate joint hyperlaxity. Muscular hypotonia and drugs such as prednisolone and D-penicillamine which alter the structure or physical properties of collagen also influence joint laxity. The determination of the relative contributions of multiple aetiological factors which influence the range of movements at a given joint represents a fascinating challenge to the clinician.

References

Ansell BM (1972) Hypermobility of joints. Mod Trends Orthop 6: 419–425

Barnett CH (1971) The mobility of synovial joints. Rheum Phys Med 11: 20–27

Beighton PH, Price A, Lord J, Dickson E (1969) Variants of the Ehlers–Danlos Syndrome. Clinical, chemical, haematological and chromosomal features of 100 patients. Ann Rheum Dis 28: 228–240

Beighton P, Horan FT (1970) Dominant inheritance of familial generalised articular hypermobility. J Bone Joint Surg [Br] 52: 145–147

Beighton PH, Solomon L, Soskolne CL (1973) Articular mobility in an African population. Ann Rheum Dis 32: 413–418

Bird HA, Tribe CR, Bacon PA (1978) Joint hypermobility leading to osteoarthrosis and chrondrocalcinosis. Ann Rheum Dis 37: 203–211

Bird HA, Wright V (1981) Traumatic synovitis in a classical guitarist: A study of joint laxity. Ann Rheum Dis 40: 161–163

Carter C, Sweetnam R (1958) Familial joint laxity and recurrent dislocation of the patella. J Bone Joint Sur [Br] 40: 664–667

Carter C, Sweetnam R (1960) Recurrent dislocation of the patella and of the shoulder. J Bone Joint Surg [Br] 42: 721–727

Carter C, Wilkinson J (1964) Persistent joint laxity and congenital dislocation of the hip. J Bone Joint Surg [Br] 46: 40–45

Finkelstein H (1916) Joint hypotonia. NY Med J 104: 942–943

Grahame R (1970) A method for measuring human skin elasticity in vivo with observations on the effects of age, sex and pregnancy. Clin Sci 39: 223–233

Grahame R, Beighton P (1969) Physical properties of the skin in the Ehlers–Danlos syndrome. Ann Rheum Dis 28: 246–252

Grahame R, Jenkins JM (1972) Joint hypermobility — asset or liability. Ann Rheum Dis 31: 109–111

Harris H, Joseph J (1949) Variation and extension of the metacarpophalangeal and interphalangeal joints of the thumb. J Bone Joint Surg [Br] 31: 547–559

Horan FT, Beighton PH (1973) Recessive inheritance of generalised joint hypermobility. Rheum Rehabil 12: 47–49

Howes RJ, Isdale IC (1971) The loose back: an unrecognised syndrome. Rheum Phys Med 11: 72–77

Key JA (1927) Hypermobility of joints as a sex linked hereditary characteristic. JAMA 88: 1710–1712

Kirk JH, Ansell BM, Bywaters EGL (1967) The hypermobility syndrome. Ann Rheum Dis 26: 419–425

Massie WK, Howarth MB (1951) Congenital dislocation of the hip. J Bone Joint Surg [AM] 33: 171–198

Moll JMH, Wright V (1971) Normal range of spinal mobility: an objective clinical study. Ann Rheum Dis 30: 381–386

Nicholas JA (1970) Injuries to knee ligaments. JAMA 212: 13: 2236–2239

Silverman S, Constine L, Harvey W, Grahame R (1975) Survey of joint mobility and in vivo skin elasticity in London school children. Ann Rheum Dis 34: 177–180

Sturkie PD (1941) Hypermobile joints in all descendants for two generations. J Hered 32: 232–234

Sutro J (1947) Hypermobility of knees due to overlengthened capsular and ligamentous tissues. Surgery 21: 67–76

Troup JDG, Hood CA, Chapman AE (1968) Measurements of the sagittal mobility of the lumbar spine and hips. Ann Phys Med 9: 308–321

Walker BA, Beighton PH, Murdoch JL (1969) The Marfanoid hypermobility syndrome. Ann Int Med 71: 349–352

Wood PHN (1971) Is hypermobility a discrete entity? Proc R Soc Med 64: 690–692

Wynne-Davies R (1970) Acetabular dysplasia and familial joint laxity. J Bone Joint Surg [Br] 52: 704–716

Wynne-Davies R (1971) Familial joint laxity. Proc R Soc Med 64: 689–690

2. Assessment of Hypermobility

A pre-requisite for the study of clinical problems associated with joint hypermobility is that adequate criteria for diagnosis and measurement should be available. In early attempts at assessment, the mobility of groups of joints was recorded to provide a simple scoring system. Subsequently, there has been a tendency to concentrate upon measurements of a single joint, but the greater precision afforded is only useful if the joint mirrors the status of the majority of other joints in the body. The evolution of precise methods is further handicapped since a particular joint that appears hypermobile, for instance an interphalangeal joint or a joint between two vertebrae, may simply be compensating for an adjacent joint that is unduly stiff. This may be either because of its anatomical structure or because of acquired disease.

There has been a gradual return towards scoring systems in which a reasonably large number of joints are assessed in a simple fashion. However, the precise degree of hyperlaxity that needs to be present before a patient can be accepted as having 'generalised joint hypermobility' remains somewhat arbitrary and at the discretion of the individual investigator, although some guidelines exist in the literature. Given that hypermobility in the majority of loose-jointed persons may be one extreme of a Gaussian distribution throughout the population, it is likely that an equal and opposite number of subjects will display generalised joint stiffness. To our knowledge, however, there has been no attempt to quantify this joint rigidity by any scoring system.

Non-mechanical Scoring Systems for Hypermobility

The first scoring system was devised by Carter and Wilkinson (1964) in conjunction with their work on congenital dislocation of the hip. They defined generalised joint laxity as being present when three of the following tests were positive, provided both upper and lower limbs were involved:

1) Passive apposition of the thumb to the flexor aspect of the forearm;
2) Passive hyperextension of the fingers so that they lie parallel with the extensor aspect of the forearm;
3) Ability to hyperextend the elbow more than 10°;

4) Ability to hyperextend the knee more than 10°;

5) An excess range of passive dorsiflexion of the ankle and eversion of the foot.

A more complex assessment was suggested by Kirk et al. (1967), but in practice this proved too time consuming for routine use. The system of Carter and Wilkinson was revised by Beighton and Horan (1969) for the measurement of joint laxity in persons with the Ehlers–Danlos syndrome (EDS). Passive dorsiflexion of the little finger beyond 90° with the forearm flat on the table was substituted for passive hyperextension of the fingers, as the latter test had proved too severe, and the range of ankle movement was replaced by forward flexion of the trunk. Patients were given a score between 0 and 5.

Grahame and Jenkins (1972) modified this system to include passive dorsiflexion of the ankle beyond 15°. In part, this was an adaptation to the subjects under study, half of whom were ballet dancers. Subsequently, Beighton et al. (1973) amended the 1969 system for use in an epidemiological survey of bone and joint disorders in a rural African Negro community in Southern Africa. They employed the same tests, but gave one point for each side of the body for the paired tests. The range of scoring was thus between 0–9, with high scores denoting greater joint laxity. The manoeuvres used in this scoring system are listed below and depicted in Figs. 2.1–2.5:

1) Passive dorsiflexion of the little fingers beyond 90° (1 point for each hand)—2 points;

2) Passive apposition of the thumbs to the flexor aspects of the forearm (1 point for each thumb)—2 points;

3) Hyperextension of the elbows beyond 10° (1 point for each elbow)—2 points;

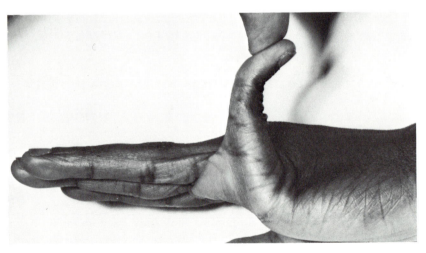

Fig. 2.1. Hyperextension of the fifth finger beyond 90°.

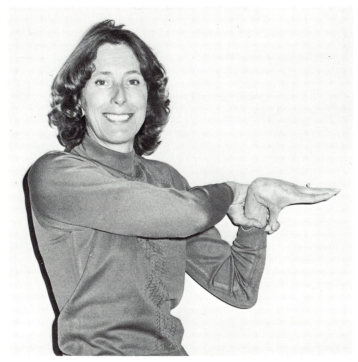

Fig. 2.2. Apposition of the thumb to the ventral aspect of the forearm.

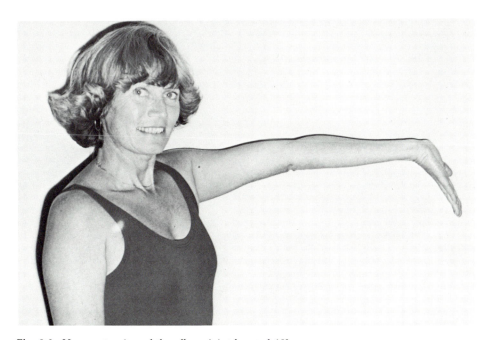

Fig. 2.3. Hyperextension of the elbow joint beyond 10°.

4) Hyperextension of the knee beyond 10° (1 point for each knee)—2 points;
5) Forward flexion of the trunk with knees fully extended so that the palms of the hands rest flat on the floor—1 point.

This method has found favour for the following reasons:

1) Scoring systems using hyperextension of the middle rather than the little finger exclude too many persons;
2) Scoring systems using ankle movements, although perhaps appropriate for dancers, are unlikely to show much variation between individuals in a normal population;
3) Scoring systems which include trunk and hip movement (composite joint movement) are more likely to reflect generalised articular laxity.

The percentage frequency distribution of mobility in 502 normal adults in the African survey is indicated by means of fitted curves in Fig. 2.6. The data show that 94% of the males and 80% of the females achieved scores of 0, 1 or 2, and this range of movement can be regarded as normal for adults in this population.

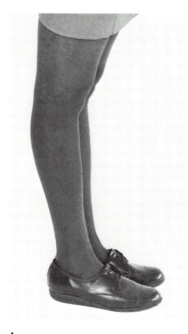

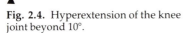

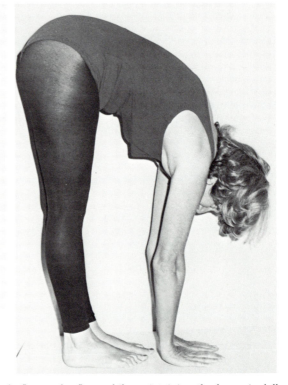

Fig. 2.4. Hyperextension of the knee joint beyond 10°.

Fig. 2.5. Placing the palms of the hands flat on the floor while maintaining the knees in full extension.

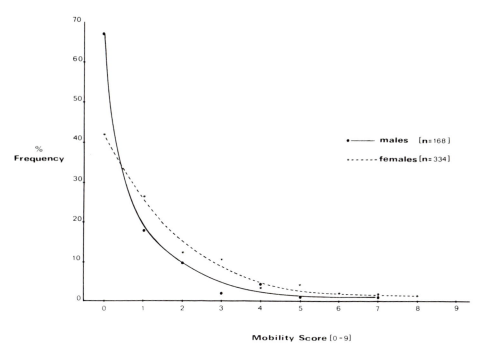

Fig. 2.6. Percentage frequency distribution of mobility score in adult South African Negroes.

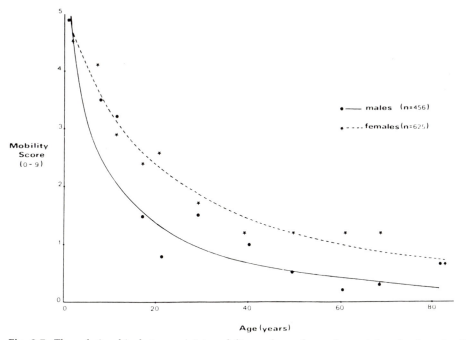

Fig. 2.7. The relationship between joint mobility and age for males and females in a South African negro population.

It is clear that the level on the scoring system at which generalised joint hypermobility is diagnosed is quite arbitrary. The majority of clinicians require a minimum score in adults of between 4/9 and 6/9 before accepting the diagnosis. However, laxity decreases with age and a lower level may be appropriate in an elderly population.

The relationship between mobility score and age, as determined in the African investigation, is shown in Fig. 2.7. At any age, females are more mobile than males. In both sexes, the degree of joint laxity diminishes rapidly throughout childhood and continues to fall more slowly in adult life.

Quantification of Hyperlaxity at Selected Joints

Little attention has been paid to the detailed measurement of movements at a single joint. The few studies undertaken have been limited in extent, since complete evaluation would require all of the following:

1) Statements on the inter- and intra-observer error of the method;
2) Consideration of the influence of age on the range of observed movement;
3) Study of sex determined differences;
4) Indication of whether specialist groups have been included in the survey population (for instance physiotherapists are often used for such studies but are likely to form a highly selective group by virtue of their training);
5) Consideration of the influence of the dominant side.

A goniometer provides the simplest method for measuring the range of movements at a hinge joint. However, there are often difficulties in positioning such an instrument and a spirit level device might be more appropriate. In this context the Loebl hydrogoniometer can be employed for determining the arc of movement at virtually any joint in the body, provided the patient is correctly positioned. Recent modifications include instruments such as the Myrin Goniometer which resemble aircraft gyro-compasses. However, this instrument lacks the sensitivity and precision of the Loebl hydrogoniometer.

Sophisticated methods are available for the appraisal of individual joints, although these are not always suitable for epidemiological studies on large populations. For instance, Harris and Joseph (1949) developed a radiological technique which they used in a study of the range of extension at the interphalangeal and metacarpophalangeal joints of the thumb in 294 subjects. Troup et al. (1968) used photography to study movement in a sagittal plane at the lumbar spine and hips. Loebl (1972) devised a mechanism for abducting the fingers to investigate movement at the metacarpophalangeal joints.

Attempts have been made to correlate goniometry with movement measured radiologically, and in these studies goniometry has frequently proved to be inadequate. The skin, fat and soft tissues may distend and cause markers on the skin to move less or more than the underlying bones. Furthermore, correlation coefficients between angular bony movement at the joint and movement of the overlying skin have rarely been provided. However, the main problem is that radiological measurements on populations are not only expensive and impractical but also unethical.

Problems with measurement of surface markers are particularly great where a group of joints move in combination, as in the lumbar spine. There is evidence that movements in adjacent joints are not equal, as some show extreme hyperextension and others slight flexion, while the overall skin pattern is that of slight extension. This has been demonstrated clearly only in cadaveric studies (Hilton et al. 1978), but the situation is likely to be similar in living subjects.

The only comprehensive account of techniques for measuring joint movement throughout the body is described in a booklet published by the American Orthopaedic Association (1965). Diagrams of suitable methods for using goniometers to determine the arcs of movement at all joints in the body are given, together with 'normal' values. However, coefficients of variation for these measurements, both between serial assessments in the same observer and between different observers, are not provided.

Mechanical Methods for Measurement of Movement at the Metacarpophalangeal Joint

The metacarpophalangeal (MCP) joint is an obvious candidate for the measurement of articular movement in large groups of persons. Not only is it a component part of conventional scoring systems, but it is also easily accessible and exhibits a wide variation in range of movement in a normal population.

Grahame and Jenkins (1972) described a simple spring device that applied a predetermined force (2 lb) to the fifth MCP joint. This preset force, applied to a relaxed patient, mimicked the passive range of movement measured in the clinical scoring system. It had good reproducibility but only quantified movement to the nearest 30°. Subsequently, the Leeds group focussed upon the problem of developing machines of greater accuracy. Those which have clinical or epidemiological application are discussed below.

Finger Hyperextensometer

The Leeds group constructed a device which would quantify hyperextension at the MCP joint of the index finger with great precision (Jobbins et al. 1979). This 'finger hyperextensometer' could be used for either hand. The results were reproducible, and the method was painless. The hyperextensometer comprises a carrier for the index finger mounted on a shaft supported by rolling element bearings (Fig. 2.8). These bearings are housed in an assembly which is fastened to a baseplate. The machine in use is depicted in Fig. 2.9.

The index finger is secured by Velcro tape to the carrier in such a way that the rotational axis of the MCP joint is in line with the axis of the operating shaft. Rotation of the joint is effected by manually turning a knurled knob and the clutch mechanism, of the spring-loaded ball type, can be set to slip at a given torque. Although the hyperextensometer is capable of applying preset torque varying between 2.0 and 7.0 kg. cm, in practice it·was found that a torque of 2.6 kg. cm was of most use in the detection of hyperlaxity in a Caucasian population.

The amplitude of rotation of the index finger at the moment of slip is indicated by a pointer fixed to the operating shaft. The finger is hyperextended and the amplitude of rotation read off from the dial. The greater the articular laxity of the subject, the greater the angle of rotation, assuming the torque remains constant.

Early studies indicated that certain precautions were necessary when using such machines. The subject had to be seated and relaxed with the elbow supported and flexed to 90°. If an individual was thought to be tense, serial measurements were taken until a plateau was reached. It was important to have the forearm parallel to the ground, but surprisingly, exact alignment of the axes of rotation of the MCP joint and the machine was not critical.

Tests of reproducibility with a single observer measuring 20 persons in random order at three different times of day showed a variation of ±2° in 19 out of 20. The variation between different operators was initially ±6°, although this figure fell as two untrained observers made successive observations. The reproducibility represented a considerable improvement on the sensitivity of existing methods.

Figure 2.10 is a scattergram showing the observed range of hyperextensometer readings in a population of 100 Caucasian individuals with normal joints. The joints of females display more hyperlaxity than their age-matched male counterparts. Values obtained from a Ghanaian male subject, a Pakistani female subject and a Turkish female subject have been added to this scattergram. It is of interest that these single examples all showed hypermobility. It is impossible to derive valid conclusions from such small numbers, but these observations may indicate that variation can occur between different ethnic groups in the range of movement at the MCP joint.

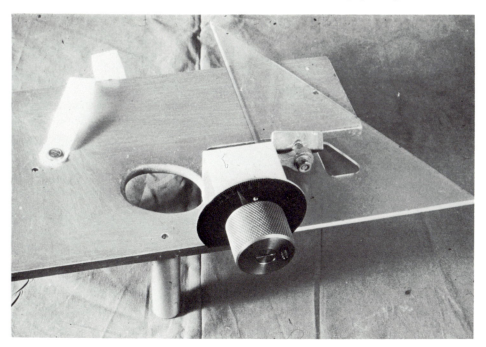

Fig. 2.8. A finger hyperextensometer for the quantification of joint laxity.

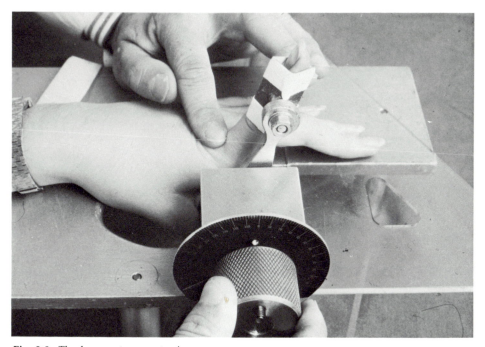

Fig. 2.9. The hyperextensometer in use.

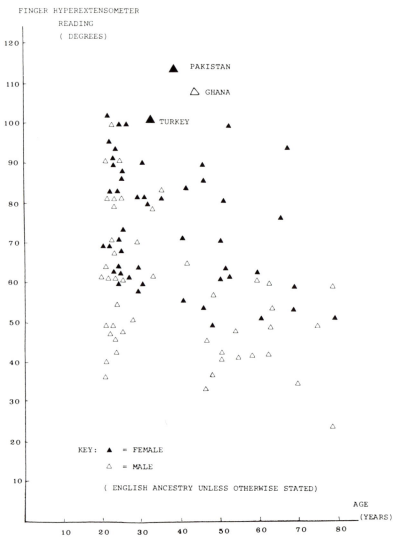

Fig. 2.10. A scattergram showing hyperextensometer readings in degrees for 100 normal persons.

Finger Arthrograph

Bird et al. (1981) constructed a finger arthrograph for the measurement of stiffness at the MCP joint. Whereas the hyperextensometer measures angular displacement in response to a preset torque, the arthrograph quantifies the resistance encountered when the index finger is moved in sinusoidal fashion at a constant speed through a pre-selected angle of displacement. The apparatus is shown in Fig. 2.11.

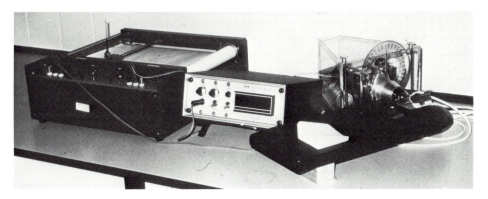

Fig. 2.11. A side view of the finger arthrograph.

The index finger is strapped by Velcro fastenings into a rotating arm, as in the finger hyperextensometer. The MCP joint is then moved through a given angular displacement by the motor (Fig. 2.12). The resistance of the joint to this movement can be recorded either as a computed digital printout or a hysteresis loop.

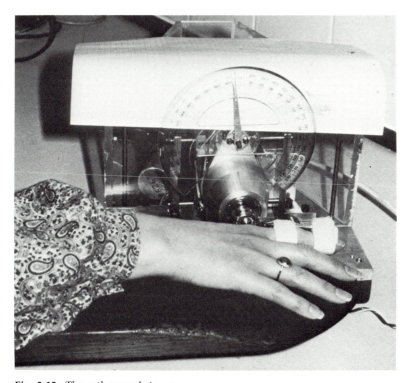

Fig. 2.12. The arthrograph in use.

Once the patient is relaxed, the motor is switched on and a hysteresis loop is recorded for each phase through which the finger is moved. It is accepted that the subject is relaxed once consecutive hysteresis loops overlap, showing that there is no active resistance to movement. This situation is normally achieved within a few seconds, but in some cases it may be necessary to leave the subject in position with the motor running for up to 2 min before relaxation is obtained.

Information on the degree of stiffness is calculated by considering either the area within the hysteresis loop or else the angle of the tangent to those parts of the loop that display maximum angular change. For example, a person with EDS and extreme hyperlaxity would have a very narrow hysteresis loop, while a patient with the shoulder-hand syndrome and pathological stiffness of the MCP joint would show corresponding widening of the loop.

In the long run, the arthrograph may provide more information concerning the components of stiffness at the MCP joints than the finger hyperextensometer. However, the hyperextensometer is a quicker and cheaper method which is better suited to epidemiological studies of large populations, and Bird et al. (1981) employed this instrument to demonstrate that slight hyperlaxity develops in the peripheral joints during pregnancy.

Evaluation of Scoring Systems Used in Assessing Joint Laxity

Three different methods of assessing joint laxity have been compared by the Leeds group. The first was the Carter and Wilkinson scoring system, as modified by Beighton et al. (1973). The second was the Leeds finger hyperextensometer (vide supra), which represented a precise assessment of laxity, albeit at a single joint. The third was a 'global index'. This was derived by using goniometry to assess the range of movement at almost all joints in the body, following the guidelines suggested by the American Academy of Orthopaedic Surgeons (1965) and summating the measured arcs of movement.

The initial survey was undertaken on students from the Carnegie School of Physical Education, Leeds Polytechnic, because it was felt that they would be interested and enthusiastic in view of their basic education in anatomy and physiology. In an attempt to consider the effects of regular athletic training upon joint hypermobility, this group was compared with age-matched non-athletic students from the same Polytechnic College. The prerequisite for entry to the control group was the playing of sport for less than half a day per week. In contrast, the physical education (PE) students devoted at least three and a half days per week to regular and varied sporting activity. In order to include as many hypermobile individuals as possible, groups of National standard swimmers and gymnasts were subsequently added and age-matched with the students at the Polytechnic.

A total of 126 individuals participated in the study. The females demonstrated more laxity than the males on all three scoring systems. It is of interest that the PE students were less lax than the non-PE students, as judged by the hyperextensometer and the global index, possibly because of the greater muscular control developed through regular physical training. The gymnasts, in particular the females, were strikingly hypermobile by all scoring systems. This finding suggests that training can serve to increase the range of movements at joints as well as stabilising them.

Correlations Between Scoring Systems

Beighton's modification to the Carter and Wilkinson system correlated well with the global index. It was easy to carry out and as quick as the hyperextensometer. Although derived on arbitrary grounds, it performed well in practice. It has been suggested by Amis (1978) that the increased carrying angle at the female elbow, which allows a greater degree of extension, might weight this scoring system in favour of females. However, the results do not bear this out. Although minor differences are seen between the right and left sides of individuals, the coarser movements measured with this system always scored equally on both sides. When both sides did not behave similarly, this was usually attributable to an earlier injury.

Overall, this system compares better than the hyperextensometer when matched against the global index. This is hardly surprising, since assessment of a single joint cannot provide as much information as appraisal of a larger number of joints. The hyperextensometer gives most information about joints of comparable anatomical structure. It may be that, although sophisticated in design, the hyperextensometer will prove unnecessarily accurate for routine use, and the Beighton modification of the Carter and Wilkinson system will be preferred for rapid assessments of the type required in population studies.

Significance of Mobility Indices

All authors agree it is easier to measure movement at a single joint than at many sites. More pertinent is whether the information obtained in this way reflects properties of joints in other regions of the body. This is clearly not so if articular disease is present. However, provided like joints are compared and the comparison is limited to joints where movement is constrained by ligaments rather than bone, the extrapolation has theoretical attractions. The correlations obtained between scoring systems in the selected populations quoted earlier in this chapter are all highly significant, suggesting that information from a single joint can indeed be extrapolated. The unanswered question, therefore, is what determinant of joint mobility the three scoring systems were measuring.

It is noteworthy that correlation coefficients were generally higher when a small group of persons who were highly selected in terms of their sporting activity, such as the gymnasts and swimmers, was analysed. This implies that the scoring systems are themselves designed to perform best on hypermobile individuals.

Determinants of Joint Mobility

Normal articular movement is a function both of the stretch of joint capsule and ligaments and of muscle tone, assuming that the tendon apparatus is mechanically intact. Animal experiments undertaken by Johns and Wright (1962) suggest that other factors, such as resistance of skin to stretch and friction within tendon sheaths, have a negligible influence upon joint mobility.

Regular training undoubtedly affects the range of movements, due either to alteration in muscle control or to stretching of the joint capsule (Fig. 2.13). Although both contribute, the former is probably much more important, though this is hard to prove. Atha and Wheatley (1976) showed the effect of training to be a source of greater variation in passive goniometry at larger joints, and it has to be specified whether the individual is 'warmed up' or participating in a physical training programme designed to increase the range of movement.

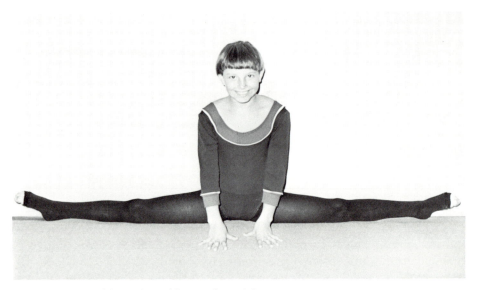

Fig. 2.13. Joint mobility achieved by regular training.

The dominant side (particularly in the hands) is likely to have more muscle tone than the less frequently used side, because of either a greater number of muscle fibres or an alteration of background intrafusal fibre afferents. This situation would be reflected in the smaller range of movement for a given force on the dominant side. This was demonstrated in epidemiological studies on a large, unselected African population by Beighton et al. (1973), but Silverman et al. (1975) found no significant differences between the two sides at the MCP joint in London schoolchildren. The choice of the population may therefore be critical. Hyperextensometer results fall between those of these two investigations.

Allocating dominance may be difficult in some persons. Indeed, it is possible that this quality is not a discrete entity and that it can be modified by occupation. For instance, a PE student in the Leeds survey could throw a javelin with his left hand, a cricket ball with his right hand and could use a pen with either!

Variation of Joint Laxity Within Populations

The range of normal joint movements decreases rapidly throughout childhood and more slowly in adulthood. This observation has been confirmed in children in Edinburgh (Wynne-Davis 1970), an African population (Beighton et al. 1973) and in British children (Silverman et al. 1975). Joint laxity continues to diminish throughout adult life (Kirk et al. 1967). The joints of females were found by several authors to be more lax than those of age-matched males (Harris and Joseph 1949; Wynne-Davis 1970; Beighton et al. 1973), though this finding has been disputed by Silverman et al. (1975).

Although no comparative studies have been carried out there is a strong clinical impression of a racial variation in joint mobility. For instance, Indians show more hyperextension of the thumb than Africans, who in turn have greater hyperextension than Europeans (Harris and Joseph 1949). A similar result has been obtained comparing the finger joints of different racial groups in Southern Africa (Schweitzer 1970). The question of inter-ethnic variation could be resolved by large scale comparative studies employing the techniques discussed in this chapter.

References

American Academy of Orthopaedic Surgeons (1965) Joint motion: method of measuring and recording Livingstone: Edinburgh
Amis AA (1978) Biomechanics of the upper limb and design of an elbow prosthesis. Ph D thesis, University of Leeds

Atha J, Wheatley DW (1976) The mobilising effects of treatment on hip flexion. Br J Sports Med 10: 22–25

Beighton PH, Horan F (1969) Orthopaedic aspects of the Ehlers–Danlos syndrome. J Bone Joint Surg [Br] 51(3): 444–453

Beighton PH, Solomon L, Soskolne CL (1973) Articular mobility in an African population. Ann Rheum Dis 32: 413–418

Bird HA, Jobbins B, Wright V (1981) A finger arthrograph for the quantification of joint stiffness. Ann Rheum Dis 40: 200–205

Bird HA, Calguneri M, Wright V (1981) Changes in joint laxity occurring during pregnancy. Ann Rheum Dis 40: 209–212

Carter C, Wilkinson J (1964) Persistent joint laxity and congenital dislocation of the hip. J Bone Joint Surg [Br] 46: 40–45

Grahame R, Jenkins JM (1972) Joint hypermobility—asset or liability. Ann Rheum Dis 31: 109–111

Harris H, Joseph J (1949) Variation in extension of the metacarpophalangeal and interphalangeal joints of the thumb. J Bone Joint Surg [Br] 31(4): 547–559

Hilton RC, Ball J, Benn RT (1978) In vitro mobility of the lumbar spine. Ann Rheum Dis 38: 378–383

Jobbins B, Bird HA, Wright V (1979) A joint hyperextensometer for the quantification of joint laxity. Eng Med 8: 103–104

Johns RJ, Wright V (1962) Relative importance of various tissues in joint stiffness. J Appl Physiol 17(5): 824–828

Kirk JA, Ansell BM, Bywaters EGL (1967) The hypermobility syndrome. Ann Rheum Dis 26: 419–425

Loebl WY (1967) Measurement of spinal posture and range of spinal movement. Ann Phys Med 9: 103–110

Loebl WY (1972) The assessment of mobility in the metacarpophalangeal joints. Rheum Phys Med 9(8): 365–379

Schweitzer G (1970) Laxity of metacarpophalangeal joints of finger and interphalangeal joint of the thumb: A comparative interracial study. S Afr Med J 44: 246–249

Silverman S, Constine L, Harvey W, Grahame R (1975) Survey of joint mobility and in vivo skin elasticity in London schoolchildren. Ann Rheum Dis 34: 177–180

Troup JDG, Hood CA, Chapman AE (1968) Measurements of the sagittal mobility of the lumbar spine and hips. Ann Phys Med 9(8): 308–321

Wynne-Davis R (1970) Acetabular dysplasia and familial joint laxity: two aetiological factors in congenital dislocation of the hip. J Bone Joint Surg [Br] 52: 704–708

3. Histopathology and Collagen Chemistry in Hypermobility

Introduction

The possible aetiology of joint hypermobility has become complicated in recent years. At one time a facile explanation sufficed; joint hyperlaxity, presumably related in some way to collagen structure, was regarded as an inherited abnormality explicable in terms of a simple, but at that stage undetermined, alteration in conventional collagen structure. However, in the last few years our understanding of hyperlaxity has increased considerably (Bird 1982), and any discussion on possible alteration of structure in hyperlax joints has to take into account the following observations:

1) The range of movement at a joint depends on several aetiological factors including the shape of the bone and cartilage (e.g. acetabular dysplasia), muscular power and tone and the laxity of the ligaments and joint capsule;

2) For any single joint, movements vary in Gaussian fashion throughout a population (Wood 1971);

3) There is probably ethnic variation;

4) Some individuals with hyperlax joints have connective tissue changes at other sites in the body which lead, for example, to floppy heart valves (Grahame et al. 1981);

5) An increasing number of discrete disorders of connective tissue such as the Ehlers–Danlos (EDS) and Marfan syndromes have been recognised. There is considerable overlap of variants of some of these conditions with familial undifferentiated joint hypermobility (Beighton et al. 1969; Walker et al. 1969);

6) There is almost certainly a wide variation between individuals in the amount of collagen at comparable sites. Studies of the collagen content of the femoral head, for example, show that this may account for between 45% and 90% of the total substance of femoral head cartilage (Kempson et al. 1970). Although our understanding of the biochemical nature of collagen continues to increase, allowance must always be made for the quantitative as well as the qualitative structure of the collagenous joint capsule.

It is clear that the possible alterations in collagen chemistry which might account for observed joint hyperlaxity are likely to be extremely complex, with considerable variation not only between individuals, but also between different sites in the same person.

Chemical Structure of Collagen

Collagen is the most important structural protein in the body, forming about 75% of the dry weight of the dermis and 50% of the weight of hyaline cartilage. Nevertheless, there is wide variation between individuals. Although synthesised within all types of connective tissue cells, collagen subsequently becomes almost entirely extracellular. The morphology is adapted to each anatomical site (Fig. 3.1.a). In tendons and ligaments where a high tensile strength is required (particularly in the former which have minimal elastin) the fibres have an orderly structure. By contrast, in cartilage the role of collagen is more of matrix reinforcement, except at the surface, where the structure becomes more dense and orderly.

Tropocollagen, the basic molecule, is rod shaped and about 30 nm long and 1.4 nm in diameter (Fig. 3.1.b). It is a triple super helix, formed from the intertwining of three polypeptides, each containing approximately 1000 amino acids (Figs. 3.1.c and d). Every third amino acid is glycine (Fig. 3.2).

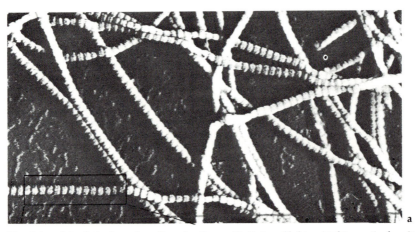

Fig. 3.1. a Metal-shadowed replica of collagen fibrils in calf skin. At this particular site the fibrils are grouped together in a lattice-like pattern that is adapted to the containing function of skin, an organ that might be stretched in any direction. In tendons the collagen fibrils would all be orientated parallel to the long axis of the tendon. The fibrils are enlarged approximately 30 000 times, the periodic spacing along a fibril being about 640 Å.

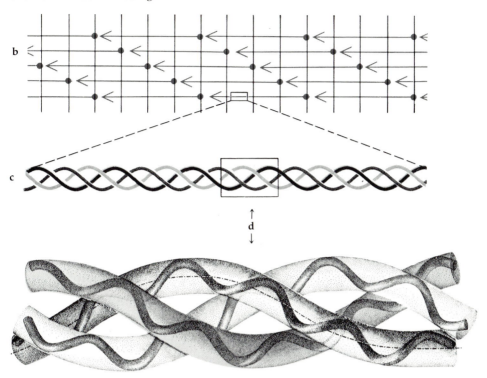

b This demonstrates in diagrammatic form the structure of one tropocollagen molecule. The area depicted is marked by a *square box* in the preceeding figure. It is believed that each tropocollagen molecule is approximately 2500 Å long and thus extends through four sets of cross-striations. In this diagram each tropocollagen molecule is represented by an arrow.

c The triple helix structure of the tropocollagen molecule. Approximately one fifth of a single tropocollagen molecule is depicted.

d A small proportion of the triple helix shown in the previous figure. Three left-handed helices are given a right-handed twist for a three-fold superhelix, thus conferring considerable strength. From Dickerson and Geis (1969).

Uncommon amino acids such as 3- and 4-hydroxyproline are present in greater concentrations than in other tissues, as is hydroxylysine. Further analysis of tropocollagen by selective cleavage into peptides has shown two further molecular species, designated a_1 and a_2, and considerable variation in the a_1 type of chain (Table 3.1). There is also a further 'fine tuning' at certain sites when after transcription by RNA, small differences may occur in proline and lysine hydroxylation and in the cleavage of N-terminal peptides. Collagen has a variable carbohydrate content, in the form of galactose and glucose covalently linked to hydroxylysine. There is a particularly large proportion of carbohydrate in the collagen of basement membrane.

Tropocollagen has a half-life of many years. The large amounts of proline and hydroxyproline together with cross-linking confer stability and resistance to many proteinases. The conversion of procollagen to collagen is mainly

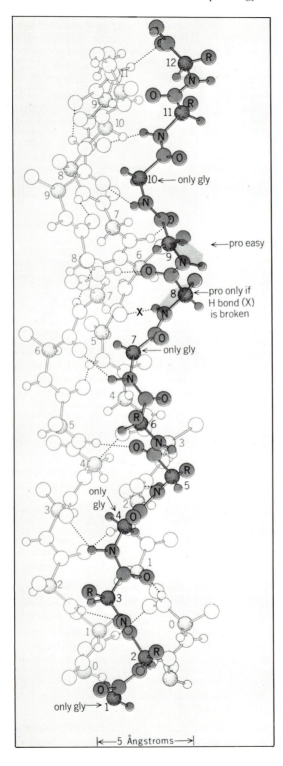

Fig. 3.2. The molecular structure of a small portion of the three-fold superhelix depicted in Fig. 3.1(d). From Dickerson and Geis (1969).

Table 3.1. Composition of tropocollagens

Type	Chain compositions	Organs in which present
I	Two α_1 (I) and one α_2 make up each triple helix.	Tendon Bone Synovium Adult skin
II	Three α_1 (II) make up each helix.	Articular cartilage Osteoid Epiphyseal growthplate
III	Three α_1 (III) make up each helix.	Synovium Foetal skin Vascular tissue
IV	Three α_1 (IV) make up each helix.	Renal glomerulus (basement membrane) Lens capsule in eye

extracellular, and requires the activity of two specific proteinases (Miller 1976). In the case of Type I collagen the $-NH_2$ terminal non-helical extension peptides are cleaved first, leaving an intermediate on which the -COOH terminal extension peptides remain intact for removal at a later stage. The axial alignment which makes up the bundles uses both ionic and hydrophobic interactions facilitated by the pitch of the superhelix approximating a value of 30–36 residues (Holmes et al. 1973; Cunningham et al. 1976). Cross-linking further stabilises the structure and is initiated by a copper-containing enzyme, lysyl oxidase.

There are two main sites for intermolecular cross-linking. Cross-links derived from precursor residues in the $-NH_2$ terminal non-helical region are formed by condensation with a hydroxylysine residue located in a helical domain near the -COOH terminal of an adjacent molecule. Further cross-links, involving precursor residues in the -COOH terminal non-helical region, are formed by condensation with a hydroxylysine residue located in a helical domain near the $-NH_2$ terminal of an adjacent molecule. Cross-linking is facilitated by an integral displacement distance so that $-NH_2$ terminals lie alongside -COOH terminals.

In the consideration of hyperlaxity, if it is accepted that an alteration in collagen may produce weakened and therefore distensible connective tissue, the sites or levels of structure at which such an abnormality may occur are many. The following hypothetical deviations of metabolism may occur:

1) The synthesis of the specific messenger-RNA for collagen may be abnormal, leading to variation in amino acid content;
2) Errors may occur at the level of transcription, leading to variation in amino acid content;
3) Variation may occur in the natural 'fine tuning' mechanism by which the amino acid content varies slightly from site to site in the same individual;

4) A defect may occur in the cleavage process that connects procollagen to collagen;

5) Variation may occur in the ionic interactions which tend to align and strengthen collagen fibres;

6) There may be a defect in cross-linking;

7) Although collagen is relatively inert, variation in the rate of metabolism of collagen may lead to quantitative rather than qualitative variation in some individuals.

Structure of Elastin

Elastic material is present throughout the body, and comprises an amorphous ground substance with a microfibrillar component. The latter is made up of the protein elastin, which consists of filaments 30–40 nm in diameter arranged in the long axis of the elastic fibres. The amino acid glycine occupies every third site on the peptide chain of elastin, reminiscent of its close association with collagen. However, the amount of hydroxyproline and hydroxylysine is reduced compared to collagen, their places being taken by unusual amino acids such as desmosine and isodesmosine, which in turn are synthesised by a copper-dependent amine oxidase. Copper deficiency therefore effectively impairs synthesis of elastin.

Desmosine, isodesmosine and lysine or leucine confer elasticity by virtue of their ability to form cross-links in the elastin polypeptide. The further microfibrillar component is rich in polar amino acids (rare in elastin) and contains no hydroxyproline, hydroxylysine or desmosine. It may confer some rigidity on the structure of elastic tissue.

The relative proportions of elastin and glycoprotein change with age, as do the appearances on electron microscopy (Giro et al. 1974). Immature and young elastic tissue retains its property of stretching, but with age it becomes increasingly calcified and rigid.

Abnormalities in collagen are more likely to account for hyperlaxity than are changes in elastin. Nevertheless there are a number of potential disturbances in elastin metabolism which may influence joint laxity:

1) A genetically determined overproduction of elastin, either in rate or amount;

2) Alterations in the amino acid content of elastin, determined on a genetic basis;

3) Premature ageing and calcification, which might hasten the loss of elastic properties.

Structure of Joints

·Bony contours and muscle tone are important in determining the degree of hyperlaxity at a joint. Indeed, it is possible that much of the 'acquired' hypermobility which may be superimposed upon genetically determined laxity may be the consequence of voluntary or involuntary alterations in muscle tone. However, the genetic contribution to hyperlaxity is most likely to reside in protein structure. Joint capsules, fascia and aponeuroses, ligaments and tendons may all be involved in determining laxity, particularly the ligaments which are endowed with a large amount of elastin. The skin and subcutaneous tissue are also important, since their extensibility is a prerequisite for a wide range of movement at joints.

The collagen in joint capsules is almost entirely Type I, and dehydroxy-lysine or leucine are the most important cross-linking compounds (Herbert et al. 1973). The structure is similar to that of tendon collagen but reduceable cross-links are virtually undetectable in individuals below the age of 20–25 years. Tendons are made from numerous collagen fibrils clustered in parallel bundles and associated with very small numbers of fibrocytes. In the largest tendons these bundles are arranged as fascicles that are separated by a small amount of loose connective tissue containing nerve fibres and blood vessels.

Ligaments are formed of dense parallel collagen bundles but contain only a limited number of fibrocytes. They are attached to bone at the enthesis (Ball 1973), where the ligamentous fibres become increasingly compact, and are fixed to bone by a cement line. A significant vascular communication exists between the ligament and the Haversian system vessels or bone marrow. This is a site of active cell metabolism and molecular exchange.

Tissue Structure in Relation to Hyperlaxity

The structure of connective tissue has been investigated by electron microscopy, which demonstrates the striated pattern of collagen fibrils, seen at a magnification of $\times 154\,000$. An interesting recent development has been the use of polarising light microscopy (Shah 1977) with a degree of resolution less than that of the electron microscope. This method shows that collagen fibrils, which may comprise many intersliding components, are mechanically coiled or 'crimped' in vitro. The wavelength of the crimp may vary between individuals or perhaps with mechanical stretching, as this 'spring' wears out with advancing age. The initial wavelength may determine the capacity of the joint for stretching in response to a given force. The preservation of the integrity of the specimen with its crimp pattern when the material is removed from the body and subjected to in vitro conditions is a considerable problem. However, there is evidence that much of the laxity of connective tissue is inherent in its physical crimp characteristics as well as in its biochemical structure.

Biochemical defects have been identified in several of the variants of the Ehlers–Danlos syndrome (EDS) (Peiris 1977; Pope et al. 1980), thus supporting the original clinical subclassification (Beighton et al. 1969; Walker et al. 1969). It is likely that other abnormalities will be recognised; for instance in EDS Type VII there may be a reduced capacity to remove the $-NH_2$ terminal procollagen extension peptides.

Investigations have been undertaken in other rare disorders of connective tissue such as hydroxylysine-deficient collagen disease (Pinnell et al. 1972; Crane et al. 1972). In this condition collagen fibrils appear morphologically normal, though dermal collagen from affected infants is more soluble than control collagen in denaturing solvents. Biochemical analysis shows a reduction in hydroxylysine content and a deficiency of enzymatic hydroxylation of lysine to collagen, which in turn results in a decreased structural integrity of this important protein. This may be the first of many inborn errors in human collagen metabolism to be defined at a biochemical level.

Although attention tends to be directed to the skin and joints as the most overt examples of hyperlaxity, variation in collagen structure at other sites may be of much greater importance to the patients. A recent preliminary communication concerning a study of polyacrylamide gel electrophoresis of skin biopsy specimens from individuals with congenital cerebral aneurysm reported that 7 out of 12 were deficient in Type III collagen (Pope et al. 1981). This was confirmed by carboxymethylcellulose chromatography of radio-actively-labelled collagens produced by cultured fibroblasts. Some cerebral aneurysms may therefore share a common aetiological pathway with the skin abnormalities seen in EDS.

Collagen in isolated floppy mitral valves has also been analysed (Bonella et al. 1980). In normal valves there was 12% cross-linked procollagen and no single-chain procollagen was found. In floppy valves these proportions were 25% and 39% respectively. The conversion of procollagen to collagen is clearly deficient, though at present it is not certain whether several or a single type of procollagen chain is involved.

There are likely to be considerable advances in our understanding of hyperlaxity in the next few years. The concept of connective tissue failure (Grahame 1969) secondary to collagen abnormality is likely to assume increasing importance with its possible association with aneurysm formation, heart valve dysfunction, hernia, pneumothorax, premature rupture of membranes in pregnancy and diverticular disease.

Alteration in Protein Structure with Disease

It has been suggested that there may be a switch in collagen synthesis from type II to type I in the cartilage once osteoarthrosis has occurred. Since type II collagen is phenotypic of cartilage, this suggests a reversion to a less differentiated state. However, the use of fluorescent antibodies specific for each type of collagen has failed to demonstrate that all type II collagen is replaced by type I collagen, and the reduced tensile strength of cartilage in osteoarthrosis in areas adjacent to the lesions that are visibly normal may be due to some other factor.

Since the bulk of our knowledge on the biochemical changes occurring in early osteoarthrosis comes from study of the Pond-Nuki dog model, in which the anterior cruciate ligament is divided to give atypical hyperlaxity, it is relevant to consider briefly the changes that may occur. It is most likely that the initial change occurs in proteoglycans (Figs. 3.3 and 3.4), which become

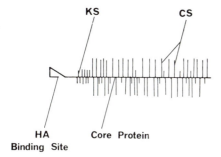

Fig. 3.3. Diagram of the manner in which the cartilage proteoglycan molecule is built up from three components, hyaluronic acid (HA), chondroitin sulphate (CS) and keratin sulphate (KS). From Muir (1977).

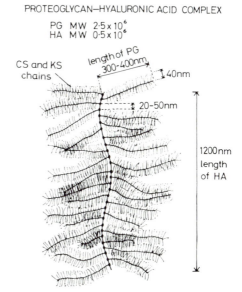

Fig. 3.4. Each cartilage proteoglycan molecule, depicted in Fig. 3.3, complexes with similar molecules at the binding site to give a 'wire brush' configuration in which the 'bristles' of each molecule splay out from a central axial chain. From Muir (1977).

more easily extracted by biochemical techniques and therefore appear to be more loosely associated with collagen compared to the proteoglycans of control cartilage. The way in which proteoglycan aggregations are built up is demonstrated in diagrammatic form (Fig. 3.5).

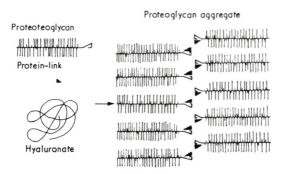

Fig. 3.5. Proteoglycan aggregation. From Muir (1977).

Action of Drugs on Collagen

Two drugs used in the treatment of rheumatic diseases, prednisolone and D-penicillamine, may also act upon collagen. In an evaluation of skin elasticity using a suction device to measure the elastic modulus and calipers to assess skin thickness, Grahame (1969) showed that in rheumatoid arthritic patients receiving prednisolone, the elastic modulus remained unaltered while skin thickness was significantly decreased. By contrast, ACTH did not cause a comparable loss of skin thickness. This observation may account for the smaller degree of steroid bruising seen in rheumatoid patients treated with ACTH rather than prednisolone. It is likely that prednisolone alters collagen in rheumatoid arthritis by changing quantity rather than quality.

The use of D-penicillamine in the treatment of scleroderma is based on a qualitative action which breaks the disulphide bridges between chains of amino acids, leading to sliding or loosening of collagen (Bluestone et al. 1970; Herbert et al. 1974). Penicillamine has also been shown in vitro to inhibit collagen synthesis by proliferating human fibroblasts (Harvey et al. 1974). The place of D-penicillamine in scleroderma is now limited to very early disease, and its value is disputed. On theoretical grounds, it might produce ligamentous laxity when high doses are prescribed, but this has not been documented in clinical practice.

References

Ball J (1973) Enthesiopathy of rheumatoid and ankylosing spondylitis. Ann Rheum Dis
30: 213–223

Beighton P, Price A, Lord J, Dickson E (1969) Variants of the Ehlers–Danlos syndrome. Clinical,
chemical, haematological and chromosomal features of 100 patients. Ann Rheum Dis
28: 228–240

Bird HA (1982) Joint and tissue laxity. In Wright V (ed) Topical reviews in rheumatic disease,
vol 2. John Wright and Sons Ltd, Bristol. In press.

Bonella D, Parker DJ, Davies MJ (1980) Accumulation of procollagen in human floppy mitral
valves. Lancet 1: 880–881

Bluestone R, Grahame R, Holloway V, Holt PJL (1970) Treatment of systemic sclerosis with
D-penicillamine. Ann Rheum Dis 29: 153–158

Crane SM, Pinnell SR, Erbe RW (1972) Lysal procollagen hydroxylase deficiency in fibroblasts
from siblings with hydroxylysine deficient collagen. Proc Nat Acad Sci USA, 69: 2899–2903

Cunningham LW, Davies HA, Hammonds RG (1976) Analysis of the association of collagen
based on structural models. Biopolymers 15: 483–502

Dickerson RE, Geis I (1969) The structure and action of proteins. Harper & Row, New York,
Evanston, London

Giro MG, Castellani I, Volpin D (1974) Elastic tissue during prenatal development. Connect
Tissue Res 2: 231–235

Grahame R (1969) Elasticity of human skin in vivo. Ann Phys Med 10: 130–136

Grahame R, Edwards JC, Pitcher D, Gabell A, Harvey W (1981) A clinical and echocardiographic
study of patients with the hypermobility syndrome. Ann Rheum Dis 40: 541–546

Harvey W, Grahame R, Toseland PA, Panayi GS (1974) In vitro effects of D(-)penicillamine on
collagen synthesis by human fibroblasts. In Peeters H (ed) Protides of biological fluids, 22nd
Colloquium. Pergamon Press, Oxford, NY, Toronto, p 75–78

Herbert CM, Jayson MIV, Bailey J (1973) Joint capsule collagen in osteoarthrosis. Ann Rheum Dis
32: 510–514

Herbert CM, Lindberg KA, Jason MIV, Bailey AJ (1974) Biosynthesis and maturation of skin
collagen in scleroderma and effect of D-penicillamine. Lancet 1: 187–192

Holmes DJS, Miller A, Parry DAD, Plez KA (1973) Analysis of primary structure of collagen for
the origins of molecular packing. J Med Biol 79: 137–148

Miller EJ (1976) Biochemical characteristics and biological significance of the genetically distinct
collagens. Med Cell Biochem 13: 165–192

Mosher DF, Schad PE, Kleinman HK (1979) Cross-linking of fibronectin to collagen by blood
coagulation factor XIIIa. J Clin Invest 64: 781–787

Muir H (1977) Heberden oration. Molecular approach to the understanding of osteoarthrosis.
Ann Rheum Dis 36: 199–209

Peiris S (1977) Ehlers–Danlos syndrome. Proc R Soc Med 70: 894–897

Pinnell, SR, Crane, SM, Kenzora J (1972) A heritable disorder of connective tissue hydroxylysine
deficient collagen disease. New Eng J Med 286: 1013–1020

Pope FM, Jones, PM, Wells RS, Lawrence D (1980) EDS IV (acrogeria). New autosomal dominant
and recessive types. J R Soc Med 73: 180–186

Pope FM, Narcissi P, Neil-Dwyer G, Nicholls AC, Bartlett J, Doshi B (1981) Some patients with
central aneurysms are deficient in Type III collagen. Lancet 1: 973–975

Shah JS, Jayson MIV, Hanson NGJ (1977) Low tension studies of collagen fibres from ligaments of
the human spine. Ann Rheum Dis 36: 139–145

Walker BA, Beighton P, Murdoch JL (1969) The Marfanoid hypermobility syndrome. Ann Int
Med 71: 349–352

Wood PHN (1971) Is hypermobility a discrete entity? Proc R Soc Med 64: 690–692

4. Biomechanics of Hypermobility; Selected Aspects

Introduction

In an early paper Sutro (1947) drew attention to the biomechanical aspects of hypermobility. In a study of recurrent effusions in the knees and ankles of USA army recruits, he noted an increased range of both active and passive movement in the affected joints. He argued in favour of an 'overlength' of certain articular, capsular and ligamentous tissues, and suggested that there might be disproportion in the relative rate of growth of the bones and their attached ligaments.

Two decades later Coomes (1962) made a detailed analysis of lateral instability of the knee joint. Movements were measured in 59 normal subjects and 57 patients with rheumatoid arthritis. Instability was present in rheumatoid patients with severely affected knee joints but not those with mild disease. Instability was not present in normal knees but adolescents up to the age of 20 displayed more lateral movement than normal adults. No change was seen in patients with ankylosing spondylitis and only moderate change in patients with psoriatic arthropathy.

Precise biomechanical studies of this type have clinical relevance, and an investigation of injuries to knee ligaments in American professional football players is of interest (Nicholas 1980). One hundred and thirty-nine players were classified as 'loose' or 'tight' and subsequently checked for the incidence of major ligament rupture requiring surgery. An increased likelihood of ligament injury was found in players with lax joints.

Mechanical Factors in Joint Mobility

Musculoskeletal

Many mechanical factors determine the range of movement at a joint. The shape of the bones is important. For instance nature requires the elbow to hyperextend, but the increased carrying angle in women allows a greater amount of hyperextension than in males. By contrast, at a ball and socket joint such as the hip or shoulder, a wide range of movement is appropriate to function and stability is achieved by muscular tone and a firm muscular collar. Movements at joints are further determined by the properties of the capsules, the ligaments and, to a lesser extent, the tendons. Finally, extensibility of the skin and subcutaneous tissue is necessary to allow articular motion.

Biochemical alterations in collagen and elastin structure may account for the inherited 'background' variation in laxity in a population and also for inter-ethnic differences. However, these molecular abnormalities, together with those rare genetic defects which produce extreme hyperlaxity, probably account for only a portion of the variation in the range of movements. A wider disparity may result from differing muscle tone which may be influenced to a significant extent by regular training or a programme of 'warming up' exercises. Logical studies to prove this point using general anaesthesia to eliminate or reduce muscle tone prior to measuring articular range have not, to our knowledge, been performed.

Articular

There are a number of theories to account for the remarkably low resistance to movement observed at synovial joints, and these may also have some bearing upon the biomechanics of hyperlaxity.

The oldest theory is that of 'hydrodynamic lubrication' first proposed by MacConaill (1932). The articular surfaces are separated by a thick film of synovial fluid. However, joint movement is too slow and the pressures across the surfaces are too high to allow the maintenance of a thick film of this nature.

Charnley (1959) postulated a mono-molecular layer of hyaluronic acid-protein complex that provides so-called 'boundary lubrication'. In the context it is noteworthy that all known bearings depending upon boundary lubrication have a coefficient of friction 20 times as high as that present in synovial joints. The synovial joint mechanism may be more analogous to 'elastohydrodynamic lubrication'. Here, rubbery surfaces are separated by films of viscous fluid.

It is likely that no single mode of lubrication can fully explain the properties of synovial joints (Dowson et al. 1981). There is clear experimental evidence of fluid film lubrication, yet mathematical analysis indicates that this mechanism is not the sole factor. Fluid films require an elastohydrodynamic entraining action supplemented by squeeze film lubrication to be effective, rather than conventional hydrodynamic action alone.

The influence of muscles and tendons is often neglected when considering the frictional forces operative at synovial joints. A tensile force is exerted by muscles and tendons in almost all positions of joints, irrespective of muscular contraction which would exert a further and more powerful force. It has been shown that joints are more mobile in their mid positions than at the extremes of their ranges (Barnett 1971). Studies on the wrist joints of dogs shortly after death show that an ever-increasing force is required to straighten the joint as the position of full extension is reached.

Soft Tissues

Most studies on the tensile properties of collagen have been carried out on tendons in the tails of rats, which can be easily freed from secondary tissue. There is little slack to take up, and the shapes of load/extension curves of collagen bundles are almost independent of the numbers of fibres which they contain.

After an initial brief alignment of the force/extension curve, there follows an essentially linear extension during which Hooke's law is obeyed. At a certain point a failure of individual fibres begins to occur until the tendon as a whole finally ruptures. Elastic fibres, by contrast, undergo appreciable extension under the action of relatively small forces, returning to their original dimensions when the force is removed. The properties of elastin are not maintained in older age groups, hence the change in the texture of normal skin in the ageing. The physical properties of skin in terms of thickness and extensibility have been studied by Grahame and Harvey (1975).

Hypermobility and Osteoarthritis

It is believed that joint hyperlaxity predisposes to premature osteoarthrosis and may even lead to pyrophosphate deposition. There are two broad explanations of this situation. Firstly, the particular collagen structure that contributes to hyperlaxity may be identical to that which leads to osteoarthrosis. In this conceptual framework the hyperlaxity is nothing more than a phenotypic marker of a certain genotype that predisposes to premature degeneration. Secondly, biomechanical factors are important in the pathogenesis of the degenerative change. In this way any hyperlaxity, however acquired, would lead to osteoarthrosis providing it fulfilled the basic biomechanical requirements. There is evidence to support both theories, and the truth may lie in a combination of the two. In favour of the biomechanical hypothesis, not all hereditary disorders of connective tissue which lead to hyperlaxity cause premature osteoarthrosis (Nuki 1982, personal communication). However, the evidence for a biomechanical pathogenesis for osteoarthrosis is equally strong.

Findings derived from the canine model of Pond and Nuki (1973) favoured the mechanical theory. Only when the cruciate ligaments had been severed did sufficient lateral instability occur to initiate the earliest chemical changes in cartilage.

The frequency with which osteoarthrosis occurs in diseases associated with joint instability is striking. The cause of the instability may be the abnormal collagen in the ligaments as in acromegaly (Grahame and Harvey 1974), or mechanical as in some neurological diseases.

The studies of the Leeds group have indicated that individuals indulging in sporting activity may be spared osteoarthrosis. It is suggested that the protective muscle tone acquired by regular training stabilises the joint and lessens the likelihood of osteoarthrosis. Surveys of professional sportsmen show that osteoarthrosis tends to develop in those who have had surgery or injuries to a joint, causing incongruity of the articulating surfaces or stretching of the ligaments. It may be significant that in a clinical and arthroscopic study of osteoarthrosis, chondrocalcinosis and joint hyperlaxity in females, no sportswomen were found to be hyperlax (Bird et al. 1978). By implication, those who indulged in regular exercise were spared the symptoms if not the actual degenerative progression.

It must be accepted that what is conventionally termed 'osteoarthrosis' is likely to be a collection of many different conditions. On this basis, hyperlaxity would seem more relevant to secondary osteoarthrosis at a small number of joints than to the primary or generalised osteoarthrosis described by Kellgren et al. (1963). The aetiology of osteoarthrosis may be analogous to the current concept of seronegative inflammatory polyarthritis where the disease occurs in the context of the appropriate genetic background, such as the HLA antigen and the relevant provocative factor, possibly infection. By analogy joint laxity could be involved in the pathogenesis of osteoarthrosis by either of these mechanisms.

Osteoarthrosis is not seen in increased frequency in obese individuals, but when it does occur it is usually worse in the medial compartment of the knee. This fact is conventionally explained by bowing of the leg and a transfer of load from the lateral to the medial compartment (Ball and Sharp 1978). The occurrence of this shift implies some ligamentous laxity, and the situation may therefore be analogous to the instability induced by cutting the cruciate ligament in the dog.

There is considerable alteration in the biomechanics following internal derangement of the knee (Frankel et al. 1971). Fractures protect joints from excessive strains (Radin 1976) and osteoarthrosis only occurs if the fracture line enters the joint cavity, leading to non-alignment of the articulating surfaces.

The concept of a mechanical aetiology of osteoarthrosis is also supported by a study which showed that in meningomyelocele, articular damage occurred only in patients who retained the power of movement (Rodnan et al. 1959). In the same way, there is low incidence of osteoarthrosis in limbs paralysed by poliomyelitis but used with the aid of supporting calipers, which eliminate unwanted lateral movement (Glyn et al. 1966).

Joint Stiffness

Stiffness of joints is important clinically. For instance, morning stiffness is a diagnostic criterion of rheumatoid arthritis while articular gelling, the subjective impression of increased stiffness after a short period of immobilisation, is well known to arthritic patients. Grip strength measurements indicate that there is a circadian rhythm both in muscle strength and in joint stiffness in normal and arthritic persons (Wright and Jones 1961).

Arthrographs have been used in the mechanical evaluation of stiffness at the metacarpophalangeal joint of the index finger. Similar instruments have also been designed for the evaluation of stiffness at the knee joint, but these are less easy to operate and patients with severe arthritis find difficulty in co-operating. However, important information has been gleaned regarding the muscular and skeletal factors that determine joint stiffness. Physiological variations noted include increased stiffness in the elderly and reduction in stiffness at higher temperatures. The arthrograph also allows distinction between the pathological stiffness that occurs in some diseases of joints, such as osteoarthrosis and rheumatoid arthritis, and the abnormal 'suppleness' in disorders of connective tissue, such as the Ehlers–Danlos syndrome.

Arthrographs have also been of use in assessing the relative importance of various tissues in determining joint stiffness. In a classic experiment using the wrist joints of anaesthetised cats, various tissues were divided in turn (Johns and Wright 1962). In the intact joint the properties were noted to be similar to those at the metacarpophalangeal joint in man. Non-linear elasticity and plasticity accounted for most of the stiffness, elasticity being twice as important as plasticity. The joint capsule contributed 47%, passive action of the muscles 41%, the tendons 10% and the skin 2% to the total torque required to move the joint in its mid-range. Towards the extremes of joint motion, the restraining effect of tendons became more important.

References

Ball J, Sharp J (1978) Osteoarthrosis. In Scott (ed) Copeman's textbook of the rheumatic diseases. Churchill Livingstone pp 595–644

Barnett CH (1971) The mobility of synovial joints. Rheum Phys Med 11: 20–27

Bird HA, Tribe CR, Bacon PA (1978) Joint hypermobility leading to osteoarthrosis and chondrocalcinosis. Ann Rheum Dis 37: 203–211

Charnley J (1959) Symposium on biomechanics, p. 12. Institution of Biomechanical Engineers, London

Coomes EN (1962) Lateral instability of the knee following polyarthritis. An experimental study. Ann Rheum Dis 21: 378–387

Dowson D, Unsworth A, Cooke AF, Guoldanovic D (1981) Lubrication of joints. Dowson, Wright
    (eds) Introduction to the biomechanics of joints and joint replacement. M.E.P. London
    pp 120–133
Frankel VH, Burstein AH, Brooks DB (1971) Biomechanics of internal derangement of the knee. J
    Bone Joint Surg [Am] 53 (5): 945–962
Glyn JH, Sutherland I, Walker GF Young AC (1966) Low incidence of osteoarthrosis of the hip
    and knee after anterior poliomyelitis: a late review. Br Med J 2: 739–742
Grahame R, Harvey W (1974) Defect of collagen in growth-hormone disorders. Lancet II: 1332
Grahame R, Harvey W (1975) Cutaneous extensibility in health and disease. Rheum Rehab
    14: 87–91
Johns RJ, Wright V (1962) Relative importance of various tissues in joint stiffness. J Appl Physiol
    17: 824–828
Kellgren JH, Lawrence JS, Bier F (1963) Genetic factors in generalised osteoarthrosis. Ann Rheum
    Dis 22: 237–255
MacConaill MA (1932) The function of intra-articular fibro cartilages, with special reference to the
    knee and inferior radio-ulnar joints. J Anat (London) 66: 210–227
Nicholas JA (1980) Injuries to knee ligaments. JAMA 212: 2236–2239
Pond MJ, Nuki G (1973) Experimentally induced osteoarthritis in the dog. Ann Rheum Dis
    32: 387–288
Radin EL (1976) Aetiology of osteoarthrosis. Clin Rheum Dis 2(3): 509–522
Rodnan GP, MacLachlan MJ, Brower TD (1959) Neuropathic joint disease (Charcot joints). Bull
    Rheum Dis 9: 183–184
Sutro CJ (1947) Hypermobility of bones due to overstrengthened capsular and ligamentous
    tissues. Surgery 21: 67–76
Wright V, Johns RJ (1961) Quantitative and qualitative analysis of joint stiffness in normal
    subjects and in patients with connective tissue diseases. Ann Rheum Dis 20: 26–31

Section II
Clinical Aspects of Hypermobility

5. Clinical Features of Hypermobility (Locomotor System and Extra-articular)

The majority of persons with lax ligaments and loose joints suffer no articular problems. For them hypermobility is a positive attribute which enables enhanced participation in a wide variety of physical activities (see Chap. 8). However not all are so fortunate, and some experience locomotor problems as a direct result of their laxity. When symptoms result, the term 'hypermobility syndrome' is applied (Kirk et al. 1967). It must be emphasised that this designation is non-specific and in this context it does not denote any precise disease entity. The spectrum of rheumatic complications in the hypermobility syndrome is wide and, in most cases, the pathogenesis of the presenting lesion is directly related to the articular laxity.

Normal 'tight' ligaments protect joints by acting as a constraint on the range of movements and by imposing stability. The lax joint lacks such safeguards, and is therefore more likely to be injured by trauma and overuse. Many of the features of the hypermobility syndrome are commonly seen in rheumatological and orthopaedic practice, but occur with far greater frequency in hypermobile individuals, as illustrated by the case histories outlined in Chap. 7.

The term 'hypermobility syndrome', as used in this chapter, pertains to all loose jointed individuals with articular symptoms. No attempt is made to distinguish between those with familial undifferentiated hypermobility and those with joint movements which are at the upper end of the normal range. This nosological problem is also discussed in Chaps. 2 and 10.

Prevalence

The true prevalence of the hypermobility syndrome in the community is unknown, but individuals with asymptomatic joint laxity certainly outnumber those who experience clinical problems. It is possible to estimate the importance of hypermobility as a cause of articular morbidity by surveying the diagnoses of patients attending rheumatology clinics. Thus, out of a sample of 9275 patients attending the rheumatology clinic at Guy's Hospital, 185 (2%) were diagnosed as suffering from the hypermobility syndrome. A similar prevalence was seen (1.7%) amongst 690 new referrals to a paediatric centre (Ansell 1972).

A significant feature of the Guy's series was the marked female preponderance. Of the 185 patients, 157 (85%) were female compared with 52% of the clinic sample as a whole. Thus, of all clinic attenders, 3.25% of the females and 0.63% of the males were considered to have the hypermobility syndrome. This female preponderance was recognised by earlier workers (Kirk et al. 1967) but had not hitherto been expressed in statistical terms.

Articular Complications

Acute Articular and Periarticular Traumatic Lesions

Acute lesions include traumatic synovitis of joints, especially of the fingers, wrists, knees and ankles, often provoked by overuse or by a fall. Tenosynovitis, torn ligaments, torn muscles, partial or complete avulsion of tendon insertions and joint capsule tears may result from overstretching. Nicholas (1970) showed that torn knee ligaments were significantly more common among hypermobile American football players than in their tight-jointed team mates.

Chronic Polyarthritis or Monoarticular Arthritis

Chronic arthritis is a common presentation of hypermobility in the rheumatology clinic, and can give rise to diagnostic difficulties. Typically there is soft tissue swelling with an effusion. This may be recurrent or persistent without the radiographic or laboratory features of inflammatory joint disease. These patients are often mistakenly diagnosed as suffering from rheumatoid arthritis. For example a hypermobile guitarist who subjected his left wrist to hyperflexion for 5 h daily while practising was thought initially to have this disease. The resultant synovitis, which impaired his playing, was eventually correctly ascribed to hypermobility (Bird and Wright 1981).

Similarly, in children, the hypermobility syndrome may mimic juvenile chronic arthritis, particularly the pauci-articular type (Bird and Wright 1978) or the polyarticular variety (Scharf and Nahir 1982). The presence of a persistent knee effusion may lead to the formation of a Baker's cyst in the popliteal fossa (Grahame 1971).

Dislocation of Joints

The loss of joint stability due to ligamentous laxity may result in recurrent dislocation after comparatively minor trauma. This is seen particularly in the patella and the shoulder. There is also an association between hypermobility of joints and congenital dislocation of the hip. A remarkable case of unilateral hip dislocation with joint laxity which was restricted to the same side has been reported by Fredensborg (1978). The occurrence of dislocations in the undifferentiated familial hypermobility syndromes is discussed in Chap. 10.

Some loose-jointed persons are able to dislocate or sublux and reduce joints at will (a feat of dubious value!). Similarly, the ability to 'crack' finger joints is sometimes a manifestation of joint laxity. The cracking results from the sudden induction of a vacuum within the distracted lax joint (Fig. 5.1).

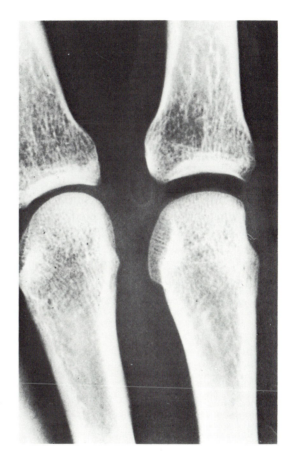

Fig. 5.1. A radiograph of a MCP joint which has been distracted and 'cracked'. The vacuum within the joint has produced a gas bubble. Reproduced by kind courtesy of Professor V Wright.

Chondromalacia Patellae

Genu recurvatum (hyperextensibility of the knee) may be an important pathogenic factor in chondromalacia patellae. There is evidence that limitation of hyperextension may reduce the symptoms of this disabling condition, which predominantly affects physically active adolescents and young adults (Walker and Schreck 1978).

Premature Osteoarthrosis

There is a strong clinical impression that hypermobility may predispose to the development of premature osteoarthrosis, particularly in weight-bearing joints. Positive proof of this hypothesis awaits controlled prospective studies. However, the widespread prevalence of osteoarthrosis in hypermobile patients, as seen in rheumatological practice, renders a pathogenetic relationship very likely, notwithstanding the influence of other important factors such as age and congenital articular dysplasia.

The additional stresses imposed upon a joint by an excessive range of movement, particularly hyperextension, and the tendency to valgus deformity of the knee and ankle that results from ligamentous laxity might well be expected to predispose to premature articular degeneration. Scott et al. (1979) compared joint mobility in a group of 50 consecutive persons aged 50 years and over with symptomatic osteoarthrosis with age and sex matched controls. These workers demonstrated a significantly higher frequency of hypermobility amongst the patients with osteoarthrosis. They conceded that hypermobility in these individuals might have been the result of the osteoarthrosis rather than vice versa, but they considered this unlikely.

Arthralgia

Joint pain, in the absence of any detectable clinical abnormality, is a frequent symptom in patients with generalised joint laxity who present to the rheumatologist. The mechanism is obscure, but many patients are able to describe aggravating and relieving factors. Changes in the climate, notably the onset of damp or cold weather, may be heralded by an exacerbation of arthralgia. The majority of female patients recognise a temporal relationship to menstruation and although many were aware of an improvement during pregnancy, a few have noted the opposite. The most consistent precipitating factor is physical activity, which is almost invariably followed by an exacerbation of joint pain. In childhood such pains are frequently described as 'growing pains', although there is no basis for this designation.

Because the pains occur in the absence of any recognisable articular abnormality, these hypermobile persons are often labelled as neurotic. This merely adds to their frustration, which stems from the failure of their medical attendants to explain or relieve their symptoms. Not surprisingly, these patients become depressed and secondary neurotic features may eventually develop.

Soft Tissue Lesions

The variety of soft tissue lesions which occur in every-day rheumatological practice seem to present with greater frequency amongst hypermobile individuals. This contention has not been tested formally, but there is a commonly-held view that this is indeed the case. Such abnormalities include tendon insertion lesions induced by overuse. Common examples are lateral and medial epicondylitis (tennis and golfer's elbow respectively), supraspinatus and bicipital tendonitis of the shoulder and adhesive capsulitis (frozen shoulder). Entrapment neuropathies may also occur in relation to a hypermobile joint. An example is the carpal tunnel syndrome in a patient with laxity of the wrist joint.

Spinal Complications

The spine, notably the lower cervical and lower lumbar regions, is commonly affected by degenerative disease in later life, as a result of the stresses to which it is submitted. This process is manifested by a combination of osteoarthrosis of the facet joints and changes in the intervertebral discs. Onset may be acute, with herniation of the nucleus pulposus through the annulus fibrosus, or chronic with osteophyte formation, leading to nerve root irritation.

It is likely that the interspinous ligaments provide an important restraining force and prevent excessive range of movement, which might otherwise lead to additional damage of the vertebrae, intervertebral discs or facet joints. It follows that a spine devoid of the protection provided by normal 'tight' ligaments will be particularly vulnerable to the insults to which the back is subjected in daily life. Thus, it is reasonable to assume that prolapse of an intervertebral disc, especially in the cervical and lumbar regions, might occur with greater frequency amongst hypermobile persons.

Fatigue fractures of the pars interarticularis (spondylolysis) with or without isthmic spondylolisthesis are also frequent in loose-jointed individuals. Notwithstanding these recognisable structural abnormalities, low back pain does seem to occur in the absence of such identifiable lesions in otherwise healthy, hypermobile subjects. This has been termed the 'loose-back syndrome' (Howes and Isdale 1971). As with arthralgia, the mechanism for the pain in this condition is unknown.

Radiological anomalies of the spine, including scoliosis, transitional vertebrae at the lumbo-sacral junction and pars interarticularis defects, with or without spondylolisthesis, are more common amongst patients with widespread joint hypermobility. Grahame et al. (1981) found that 73% of a series of 15 patients with a hypermobility score of greater than 5 showed such anomalies compared with only 33% of a matched group with a score of 3–4 and 23% of those with a score of 0–2. The differences between the first group and the others were statistically significant.

An attempt to correlate the development of spondylolisthesis with joint laxity amongst 364 female teachers of physical education failed to produce a significant result (Bird et al. 1980). However, this negative finding may have been due to the fact that the information was elicited by means of a postal questionnaire. Nevertheless, a higher prevalence of concomitants of joint laxity, such as flat feet, was recorded amongst the hypermobile subjects. It is of interest that the spondylolisthesis which occurred in this group was, with a single exception, exclusively of the degenerative (pseudo-spondylolisthesis) rather than the isthmic variety.

Idiopathic Protrusio Acetabuli

In a series of eight children aged 9 to 15 years, with progressive idiopathic protrusio acetabulae six were hypermobile (Shore et al. 1981). It is difficult to know whether the joint laxity was a primary or secondary phenomenon in these cases.

Bone Fragility

Some hypermobile persons may have a bone defect which predisposes to fracture. Thus, in a series of 33 patients with a hypermobility score of 5–9, 17 (52%) gave a past history of fracture compared with only 14% of a matched group with a hypermobility score of 3–4 and 15% of a control group with a score of 0–2 (Grahame et al. 1981). These findings suggest that there might be a common collagen defect of ligaments and bone in patients with the hypermobility syndrome. By contrast, there was no excess of fractures in a series of 100 patients with the Ehlers–Danlos syndrome (EDS) (Beighton and Horan 1969). This discrepancy might reflect differences in the nature and distribution of the fundamental abnormalities of connective tissue in these disorders.

Acquired Hypermobility

Acquired hypermobility implies an excessive range of movement occurring in one or more joints as a result of a pathological process. This laxity may be isolated or generalised.

Isolated Acquired Hypermobility

Acquired hypermobility confined to a single joint is seen in its most spectacular form in neuropathic arthropathy (Charcot's joint). Lesser degrees are encountered, commonly in rheumatoid arthritis and related diseases, where increased laxity as a result of destruction of joint surfaces may lead to subluxation and deformity. Traumatic rupture of ligaments, such as the collateral and cruciate ligaments of the knee, may also give rise to an exaggerated range of joint movement in a particular direction.

Generalised Acquired Hypermobility

Acromegaly

Polyarticular acquired hypermobility is seen in acromegaly, where principally the spine is involved. The excessive range of movement is presumably the result of hypertrophy of the intervertebral discs, together with laxity of the hypertrophic paraspinal ligaments. Thus, in a series of 42 acromegalic patients compared with control subjects (Bluestone et al. 1971), spinal movements were increased in terms of the finger-floor distance (a composite measure of spinal plus hip movements). This relative hypermobility was present in the acromegalic individuals despite gross radiological degenerative changes throughout the spine. There was, however, no clear correlation between the locomotor changes and the effectiveness of treatment of the acromegaly. Unfortunately, these authors did not report on the mobility of peripheral joints in these patients.

Studies on the tensile properties of human skin in vivo provide a rational basis for the ligamentous laxity seen in acromegaly (Grahame and Harvey 1974). In 30 acromegalic persons there was significant lowering of the elastic modulus compared with matched controls, but there was no significant correlation between the modulus and either plasma growth-hormone or the heelpad thickness. Interestingly, a group of patients with hypopituitarism showed the opposite effect, having a raised modulus of elasticity. These results suggest that collagen defects may occur in growth-hormone disorders, although their biochemical basis remains to be elucidated.

Rheumatic Fever

Rheumatic fever has been reported as producing hypermobility in the fingers of juvenile patients (Callegarini 1957). However, a subsequent study failed to confirm this finding (Kirk et al. 1967).

Hyperparathyroidism

Laxity of joint capsules and ligamentous structures has been described in hyperparathyroidism (Persellin and Rutstein 1979). This abnormality is believed to be due to the effect of parathormone, which increases collagenase activity (Stern et al. 1965). A variety of complications have been encountered, including tendon ruptures (Preston and Adicoff 1962), cervical vertebral sub-luxation, intervertebral disc protrusion and degenerative lumbar spinal disease.

Chronic Alcoholism

Widespread hypermobility of joints has been recognised in a Swedish investigation of 24 women with chronic alcoholism, compared with suitably matched controls (Carlsson and Rundgren 1980). Using the criteria of Carter and Wilkinson the authors reported the mean number of hypermobile joints as 6.30 ± 2.39 in the alcoholic patients compared with 1.05 ± 1.03 in the controls ($P < 0.01$). Articular laxity was most pronounced in the hands and least in the knees, and there were no differences in the hypermobility scores in those alcoholics with abnormal as opposed to normal liver function tests. The authors assumed that the hypermobility was acquired, and associated with the misuse of alcohol. Whether it was due to a direct effect of alcohol or its metabolites on connective tissue or secondary to liver damage leading to altered hormonal metabolism could not be determined.

Hypermobility and the Arthritides

Hypermobile subjects are not precluded from suffering from other rheumatic disorders. Indeed, when they do become thus afflicted, their pre-existing generous range of joint movement often mitigates the adverse effects of the acquired disease on articular mobility.

Ankylosing Spondylitis

Loss of spinal mobility in ankylosing spondylitis may pass unnoticed in patients with hypermobile spines, thereby delaying the establishment of the correct diagnosis (Bird 1979).

Rheumatoid Arthritis

In rheumatoid arthritis, the reduction of joint movement may be more than compensated by pre-existing hypermobility. The effects of certain deformities may also be modified. For example, patients with rheumatoid arthritis cannot normally voluntarily overcome hyperextension of the proximal interpha-langeal joints in the swan-neck deformity of the fingers. However, persons with inherent joint laxity who subsequently develop rheumatoid arthritis with this deformity may retain the ability to overcome the hyperextension and thereby enjoy good hand function, which they would otherwise have lost (Figs. 5.2 and 5.3).

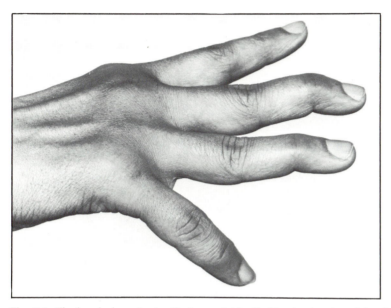

Fig. 5.2. The hand of a patient with rheumatoid arthritis who developed the classical swan-neck deformity of her fingers.

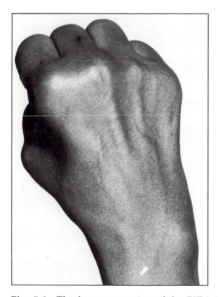

Fig. 5.3. The hyperextension of the PIP joints which is depicted in Fig. 5.2 can be overcome by virtue of inherent ligamentous laxity.

Osteoarthrosis

It is not known whether all hypermobile persons who develop osteoarthrosis in their lax joints suffer more severe symptoms. However, there seems no doubt that extreme forms of osteoarthrosis may result when multiple sequelae of hypermobility co-exist and interact (Fig. 5.4).

As a general rule, hypermobility decreases with age, with a consequent reduction in some of the sequelae of osteoarthrosis such as joint pain.

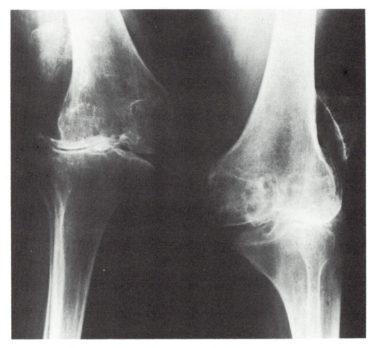

Fig. 5.4. Radiograph of the knee joint of a hypermobile adult showing gross osteoarthrosis associated with chronic dislocation of both patella and marked genu valgum, which is accentuated on weight bearing.

Non-articular Manifestations of Hypermobility

Cardiovascular System

Mitral Valve Prolapse

Mitral valve prolapse (MVP) during systole has been reported in patients suffering from hereditary disorders of connective tissue such as the Marfan syndrome (Popock and Barlow 1971; Brown et al. 1975), EDS (Brandt et al. 1975; Cabeen et al. 1977) and osteogenesis imperfecta (Woods et al. 1973). MVP is believed to be due to the presence of defective or deficient collagen in the mitral valve leaflets, leading to leaflet expansion and chordal elongation. An increase in procollagen has been found in the mitral valve of some individuals with MVP (Bonella et al. 1980).

An increased prevalence of mitral valve prolapse in persons with hypermobility has also been recorded (Grahame et al. 1981). This latter investigation was concerned with the cardiological and echocardiographic findings in three matched groups of patients with hypermobility scores 5–9, 3–4 and 0–2 respectively (Fig. 5.5).

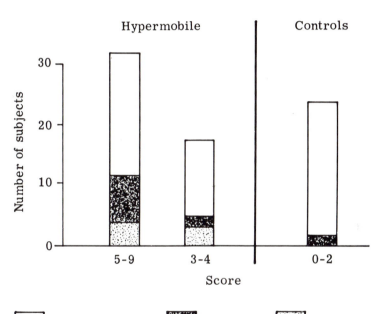

Fig. 5.5. Histogram showing mitral value prolapse amongst hypermobility syndrome patients and controls. Reproduced by kind permission of the editor and publisher.

In a further investigation Pitcher and Grahame (1982) have conducted a comparative study of 21 patients with MVP and a control group matched for age, sex and mode of presentation but without clinical or echocardiographical evidence of MVP. Hypermobility of joints was significantly more common in the MVP group, being present in 7 out of 21 patients compared with only 1 out of 21 controls ($P < 0.05$). These results provide further evidence of an association between MVP and hypermobility which is presumably due to a defect of connective tissue common to both joints and valves.

Aortic Wall Compliance

Compliance of the aortic wall is a parameter of the tensile properties of connective tissue and can be estimated by non-invasive methods. Continuous wave Doppler ultrasound measurements of pulsewave transit time between the left subclavian artery and the abdominal aorta have revealed a significant delay, denoting increased aortic wall compliance or distensibility, in patients suffering from the Marfan syndrome and several types of EDS (Child et al. 1981).

Preliminary results of a study of aortic wall compliance in hypermobility patients are available (Child and Grahame, unpublished data). Thirteen females aged 12–72 years were investigated and elevated aortic compliance values were found in nine (Fig. 5.6). These abnormal values ranged from 134% to 217% of normal (normal values of 80%–120% represent the mean values ±2 standard deviations) and were similar to those found in the Marfan and Ehlers–Danlos syndromes. These data lend further evidence to the hypothesis that hypermobility may be the consequence of a primary disorder of connective tissue.

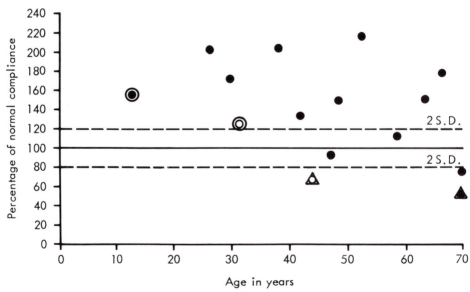

Fig. 5.6. Aortic compliance levels in 13 persons with the hypermobility syndrome. Members of the same family are indicated by similar symbols. Normal values ±2 SD are 80%–120%, based upon a volunteer population of 900 subjects of all ages and both sexes.

Changes in Joint Laxity During Pregnancy

Abramson et al. (1934) demonstrated radiologically that relaxation of the symphysis pubis occurs in pregnancy. This begins in the first trimester and increases during the last 3 months. The subsequent return to normal commences soon after delivery and is complete within 3–5 months. Zarrow et al. (1955) showed that these changes correlate with the levels of the hormone relaxin which increase tenfold during pregnancy, reaching a maximum at 38–42 weeks after conception. However, it is possible that other hormones, including progestogens and endogenous cortisol, may also play a part.

A study by Bird et al. (1981) quantified peripheral joint laxity in a group of 68 females both during pregnancy and after delivery, each subject acting as her own control. The mean age of this group was 27.16 years (range 18–40 years) and 35 were primigravidae and 33 multigravidae. Assessments were made using both the Beighton modification of the Carter and Wilkinson scoring system and the finger hyperextensometer. A first assessment was performed on each subject between the 24th and 40th week of pregnancy (mean 33.0 weeks) at a routine antenatal clinic visit. A second assessment was performed on each individual, usually at home, between 5 and 25 weeks after delivery (mean 15.1 weeks). It was anticipated that by this stage hormone levels would have reverted to normal.

Since laxity diminishes with age, the population was divided into five cohorts (less than 22 years; 22–25; 26–28; 29–31; 32 or greater). Analysis by both methods after delivery for each of these four sets showed that there was absolutely no detectable difference between them that could be attributed to age. Thereafter, the population was regarded as a single homogeneous group.

Although the modified Carter and Wilkinson scoring system failed to detect any significant difference, the finger hyperextensometer recorded a small but highly significant increase in laxity occurring during pregnancy. Hyperextension at the metacarpophalangeal joints was then analysed in relation to the number of previous pregnancies. Although there was some increase in hyperextension in primigravida, this was much more marked in women experiencing their second pregnancies. By contrast, there was little further increase in laxity in a third or fourth pregnancy.

The hypothesis that inherited hyperlaxity might be related to lack of formation of abdominal striae after delivery was also considered. Little evidence to support this theory was found, 41 subjects displaying striae and 27 subjects having none. There was no significant difference in the mean hyperextensometer reading between these groups either during or after pregnancy.

Changes in the pelvic joints during late pregnancy may arise from both local and systemic causes. The former include the weight of the gravid uterus upon the pelvic brim while the latter are presumably circulating hormones. Assessment of laxity at a peripheral joint permits separation of these factors. No previous studies on peripheral joints during pregnancy are known, apart from a relatively subjective study on ligamentous instability in the knee occurring in women after childbirth (Klein 1972). This is therefore the first study to demonstrate a clear alteration in the laxity of peripheral joints during pregnancy, though whether this finding should be attributed to relaxin, progestogens and oestrogens or altered steroid metabolism remains to be determined.

Habitus

Hypermobile patients attending the Guy's Hospital rheumatology clinic who lacked evidence of any overt hereditary connective tissue condition showed a tendency to a marfanoid habitus. Amongst these a significantly higher proportion of those with more severe generalised hypermobility had an upper segment–lower segment ratio that was within the marfanoid range (Fig. 5.7). This finding could be interpreted as supporting the hypothesis that the so-called hypermobility syndrome may be a *forme fruste* of an hereditary disorder of connective tissue, rather than representing the upper limit of a normal Gaussian distribution of joint mobility (Grahame et al. 1981).

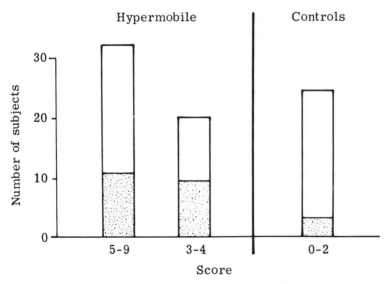

Fig. 5.7. Histogram showing a reduced upper segment/lower segment ratio in matched groups of hypermobility syndrome and control patients. Reproduced by kind permission of the editor and publisher.

References

Locomotor System Complications

Ansell BM (1972) Hypermobility of joints. Mod Trends Orthop 6: 419–425

Beighton P, Horan (1969) Orthopaedic aspects of the Ehlers–Danlos syndrome. J Bone Joint Surg [Br] (3): 444–453

Bird HA, Tribe CR, Bacon PA (1978) Joint hypermobility leading to osteoarthrosis and chondro-calcinosis. Ann Rheum Dis 37: 203–211

Bird HA, Wright V (1978) Joint hypermobility mimicking pauciarticular juvenile chronic arthritis. Br Med J 3: 402–403

Bird HA (1979) Joint hypermobility. MD Thesis, University of Cambridge

Bird HA, Hudson A, Eastmond CJ, Wright V (1980) Joint laxity and osteoarthrosis: a radiological survey of female physical education specialists. Br J Sports Med 14 (4): 179–188

Bird HA, Eastmond CJ, Hudson A, Wright V (1980) Is generalised joint laxity a factor in spondylolisthesis? Scand J Rheum 9: 203–205

Bluestone R, Bywaters EGL, Hartog M, Holt PJL, Hide S (1971) Acromegalic arthropathy. Ann Rheum Dis 30: 243–258

Callegarini U (1957) Clinical study on the hyperextensibility of fingers in rheumatic children. Bull St Francis Hosp New York 14: 32–36

Carlsson C, Rundgren A (1980) Hypermobility of the joints in women alcoholics. J Stud Alcohol 41 (1): 78–81

Fredensborg N (1978) Unilateral joint laxity in unilateral congenital dislocation of the hip. Orthop 2 (2): 177–178

Grahame R (1971) Joint hypermobility—clinical aspects. Proc Soc Med 64:692–694

Grahame R, Harvey W (1974) Defect of collagen in growth-hormone disorders? Lancet 2: 1332

Grahame R, Edwards JC, Pitcher D, Gabell A, Harvey W (1981) A clinical and echocardiographic study of patients with the hypermobility syndrome. Ann Rheum Dis 40: 541–546

Howes RJ, Isdale IC (1971) The loose back: an unrecognised syndrome. Rheum Phy Med 11: 72–77

Kirk JA, Ansell BM, Bywaters EGL (1967) The hypermobility syndrome. Ann Rheum Dis 26: 419–425

Nicholas JA (1970) Injuries to knee ligaments. JAMA 212 (13): 2236–2239

Persellin RH, Rutstein RE (1979) In McCarty DJ (ed) Rheumatic aspects of endocrinopathies in arthritis and allied conditions, 9th edn. Lea and Febiger, Philadelphia: 1326

Preston FN, Adicoff A (1962) Hyperparathyroidism with avulsion of 3 major tendons. New Eng J Med 266: 968–971

Scharf Y, Nahir AM (1982) Hypermobility syndrome mimicking juvenile chronic arthritis. Rheum Rehab 21: 78–80

Scott D, Bird HA, Wright V (1979) Joint laxity leading to osteoarthrosis. Rheum Rehab 18: 167–169

Shore A, Macauley D, Ansell BM (1981) Idiopathic protrusio acetabuli in juveniles. Rheum Rehab XX (1): 1–10

Stern BD, Glincher MJ, Mechanic GL (1965) Proc Soc Exp Biol Med 119: 577

Walker HL, Schreck RC (1978) Relationship of hyperextended gait pattern to chondromalacia patellae. Physiotherapy 1: 8–9

Extra-articular Manifestations

Abramson D, Roberts SM, Wilson PD (1934) Relaxation of the pelvic joints in pregnancy. Surg Gynaecol Obstet 58: 595–613

Bird HA, Calguneri M, Wright V (1981) Changes in joint laxity occurring during pregnancy. Ann Rheum Dis 40: 209–214

Bonella D, Parker DJ, Davies MJ (1980) Accumulation of procollagen in human floppy mitral valves. Lancet 1: 880–881

Brandt KD, Sumner RD, Ryan TG, Cohen AS (1975) Herniation of mitral valve leaflet in the Ehlers–Danlos syndrome. Am J Cardiol 36: 524–528

Brown OR, Demots H, Kloster JE, Roberts A, Menasche VD, Beals RK (1975) Aortic root dilatation and mitral valve prolapse in Marfan's syndrome. Circulation 52: 651–657

Cabeen WR, Reza MF, Kovick RB, Stern MS (1977) Mitral valve prolapse and conduction defects in Ehlers–Danlos syndrome. Arch Int Med 137: 1227–1231

Child AN, Dorrance DE, Jay B, Pope FM Jones RB, Gosling RG (1981) Aortic compliance in connective tissue diseases affecting the eye. Ophthal Pediat Genet 1(1): 59–76

Grahame R, Edwards JC, Pitcher D, Gabell A, Harvey W (1981) A clinical and echocardiographic study of patients with the hypermobility syndrome. Ann Rheum Dis 40: 541–546

Klein K (1972) The effect of parturition on ligament stability of the knee in female subjects and its potential for traumatic arthritic change. Ann Correct Ther J 26: 43–45

Pitcher D, Grahame R (1982) Mitral valve prolapse and joint hypermobility: evidence for systemic connective tissue abnormality. Ann Rheum Dis 41: 352–354

Popock WA, Barlow JB (1971) Aetiology and electrocardiographic features of the billowing posterior mitral leaflet syndrome: analysis of a further 130 patients with a late systolic murmur or non-ejection systolic click. Am J Med 51: 73–78

Woods SJ, Thomas J, Brainbridge NV (1973) Mitral valve disease and open heart surgery in osteogenesis imperfecta tarda. Br Heart J 35: 103–106

Zarrow M, Holstrom EG, Salhanick HA (1955) The concentration of relaxin in the blood serum and other tissues of women during pregnancy. J Clin Endocrinol 15: 22–27

6. Management of Articular Complications in the Hypermobility Syndrome

Hypermobile patients can be spared much unnecessary suffering by establishment of the correct diagnosis. As indicated in Chap. 5, hypermobility is one of the great mimics in rheumatology. Many hapless individuals have been misdiagnosed as suffering from rheumatoid arthritis (both adult and juvenile) with unfortunate consequences. It is self-evident that reassurance to the patient that he or she does not have a potentially crippling disease can have a profoundly beneficial effect on morale!

General Management

Although the precise cause of pain in the hypermobility syndrome is often undetermined, most patients can offer information concerning exacerbating and relieving factors. The majority recognise the adverse effects of physical activity and it is often possible to restrict exercise to within reasonable levels of tolerance. This may entail avoidance of strenuous sporting pursuits, change of occupation, or modification of the manner of performance of a particular job. The journey to and from the place of employment may provoke more symptoms than the actual work itself. In this respect time spent in taking a detailed history will pay dividends.

Specific Management

The reader is recommended to consult the standard texts of rheumatology and orthopaedics for a full account of the management of the wide variety of complications that may be associated with joint hypermobility. A summary of the principal methods is given below.

Local Steroid Injection

The treatment of choice in many of the soft tissue lesions associated with hypermobility is the careful topical infiltration with hydrocortisone acetate and lignocaine. These entities include tennis and golfer's elbow (lateral and medial epicondylitis respectively), bicipital and supraspinatus tendonitis, adhesive capsulitis, tenosynovitis, bursitis and ligamentous and capsular tears. Longer acting corticosteroid preparations should not be used in these extra-articular complications, as they may lead to severe connective tissue atrophy with consequent weakening of collageneous tissues. The injection of steroid directly into a tendon should be avoided.

A small volume of a potent steroid preparation, such as methyl predniso-lone or triamcinolone hexacetonide, gives excellent results in the treatment of persistent synovitis of joints and of the carpal tunnel syndrome. In the treatment of discogenic sciatica or cruralgia, epidural corticosteroid injections bring relief in over two-thirds of cases, whether or not hypermobility is a predisposing factor (Dilke et al. 1973).

Physiotherapy

Fashions in physiotherapy wax and wane. The last decade has seen a decline in the use of exercise therapy in the United Kingdom and elsewhere, with an upswing in the employment of procedures involving ultrasound and passive mobilisation (Maitland 1977). At therapeutic levels ultrasound has been shown experimentally to promote in vitro collagen synthesis by human fibroblasts (Harvey et al. 1975). The clinical application of this technique in the hypermobility syndrome lies in the treatment of traumatic lesions of ligament and muscle. It is also used in disorders of attachment of tendon to bone such as tennis and golfer's elbow, but is generally not as effective as local corticosteroid injection in these conditions.

Passive mobilisation is widely used in the treatment of adhesive capsulitis of the shoulder and of cervical spondylosis in the absence of cord or nerve compression. It is also employed for low back pain which is not due to bony pathology or disc prolapse with nerve or cord compression. A word of caution is needed as regards the use of forceful manipulation in hypermobile patients, as joint subluxation may result from over-enthusiasm! Gentle mobilisation procedures, however, are very useful, particularly in those individuals in whom degenerative changes in the facet joints cause trouble-some locking. Although exercise therapy has been widely used in the treatment of back pain, the value of this technique has appeared unconvinc-ing in recent trials (Davies et al. 1979; Coxhead et al. 1981).

Acute back pain in hypermobile subjects who 'over-stretch' almost certainly results from torn muscles or ligaments in the lumbar region, although more serious damage to the vertebral body, neural arch, or intervertebral disc may occur. The temporary use of a supporting lumbo-sacral surgical corset is often extremely helpful. Where pain and muscle spasm are severe, a period of rest in bed should be recommended. Traction has little, if any, role in the treatment of cervical or lumbar pain in the hypermobility syndrome and indeed may be harmful.

A problem that commonly confronts hypermobile subjects is peripheral articular instability, especially of the weight-bearing joints. This is usually the result of ligamentous tears that have occurred as a consequence of pre-existing laxity. The ankle joint is especially vulnerable. Attention to the torn ligament is only part of the management of such conditions, and it is essential to improve the stability of the joint by appropriate muscle strengthening exercises. However, care must be taken to avoid hyperextension of a lax knee with strenuous and uncontrolled quadriceps exercises, as this merely aggravates the condition. Synchronous isometric contraction of the quadriceps muscles and their antagonists should be carried out; this is particularly important when treating chondromalacia patellae, which is frequently seen in hypermobile subjects and for which physiotherapy is often prescribed.

Surgical Intervention

Certain complications of hypermobility require surgical measures, usually after conservative treatment has failed to relieve the problem. The following categories are encountered:

Soft tissue lesions such as tennis and golfer's elbow, tendonitis of the shoulder and the carpal tunnel syndrome may need operation. Tenosynovitis which has failed to respond to repeated treatment with local corticosteroid injections and other measures will very occasionally require surgical management.

Persistent synovitis in a joint which has failed to respond to local steroid injections may require a surgical synovectomy. Alternatively, if the patient is over 45 years of age, a radiation synovectomy by means of intra-articular injection of yttrium 90 or other suitable isotope may be employed. Radiation synovectomy carries a risk of causing leakage of radioactive material from the joint with consequent exposure of the inguinal lymph nodes to ionising radiation. However, this problem has not received special attention in hypermobile persons.

Recurrent dislocation of the patella, shoulder or other joint may require stabilisation to obviate further dislocation.

Cervical or lumbar laminectomy may be indicated to remove a prolapsed intervertebral disc. When instability occurs as in isthmic spondylolistheses, spinal fusion may be necessary.

Advanced osteoarthrosis of the hip or knee complicating hypermobility may require total joint replacement, as in patients without hypermobility. Pain is a major consideration in determining whether such a procedure should be undertaken, as mobility is likely to be less impaired than in non-hypermobile persons.

Symptomatic Treatment

Many of the complications in the locomotor system of patients with the hypermobility syndrome can be attributed to clearly designated local lesions. Specific treatment, if appropriately applied, provides a satisfactory remedy. Many patients, however, suffer from arthralgia and/or back pain for which no overt identifiable cause is discernible. Trigger mechanisms may be recognised and, where possible, removed. For many patients, however, the only solution lies in symptomatic pain relief, as described below.

Analgesic and Non-steroidal Anti-inflammatory Drugs (NSAIDs)

Pure analgesic drugs, such as paracetamol, dextroproxyphene and dihydrocodeine are helpful in relieving mild musculo-skeletal pain. However, many patients prefer the NSAIDs, which seem to have a propensity to relieve locomotor system pain whether in joint, bone, tendon, ligament or muscle. A wide variety of drugs are available:

1) Salicylates—aspirin in various forms;
2) Pyrazoles—phenylbutazone, oxyphenbutazone, azapropazone;
3) Indene derivatives—indomethacin, sulindac;
4) Propionic acid derivatives—naproxen, ketoprofen, fenoprofen, ibuprofen, indoprofen, fenbufen
5) Aryl-acetic acid derivatives—diclofenac, fenclofenac
6) Oxicam derivatives—piroxicam

All these drugs are capable of causing skin rashes and gastrointestinal intolerance, and the possible risk of side-effects should be weighed against the need for analgesia. It is important to re-emphasise that drug therapy is not indicated for a lesion which requires local treatment only. Medicinal agents, however, can provide a satisfactory level of analgesia for hypermobile patients with intractable arthralgia and/or back pain.

Hydrotherapy and Water Immersion

Many patients derive symptomatic pain relief from hydrotherapy, in which exercises are performed under the supervision of a physiotherapist in a pool warmed to a temperature of 35°C. Indeed, some appear to gain more benefit from immersion in the pool than from the exercises. This apparent benefit may have a rational basis (Grahame et al. 1978). If a hydrotherapy pool is not available, patients can be advised to soak at leisure in a warm bath.

Acupuncture and Transcutaneous Neural Electrical Stimulation

The use of electrical stimulation to relieve pain dates back to Ancient Greece where the electric torpedo fish was prescribed for headaches and arthritis. Acupuncture is of equally ancient derivation.

A small number of hypermobile patients have recently derived considerable relief from arthralgia through treatment with acupuncture. The formulation of the 'gate control theory' (Melzak and Wall 1965) has contributed to our knowledge of pain relief, but it is clear that further studies are needed to assess the role of these techniques in the treatment of intractable pain.

References

Coxhead CE, Inskip H, Mead TW, North WRS, Troup JDG (1981) Multicentre trial of physiotherapy in the management of sciatic symptoms. Lancet 1: 1065–1068

Davies J, Gibson T, Tester L (1979) The value of exercises in the treatment of low back pain. Rheum Rehab 18: 247–252

Dilke TFW, Burry HC, Grahame R (1973) Extradural corticosteroid injection in the management of lumbar nerve root compression. Br Med J 265–267

Grahame R, Kitchen S, Hunt J (1978) The diuretic, natriuretic and kaliuretic effects of water immersion. Quart J Med 45: 579–585

Harvey W, Dyson M, Pond JB, Grahame R (1975) The 'in vitro' stimulation of protein synthesis in human fibroblasts by therapeutic levels of ultrasound. Proceedings of the 2nd European Congress on Ultrasonics in Medicine. Excerpta Medica, Amsterdam, Oxford

Maitland GD (1977) Vertebral manipulation, 4th edn. Butterworth, London

Melzak R, Wall P (1965) Pain mechanisms. Science 150: 971–975

7. Illustrative Case Histories

The following case histories have been drawn from the records of patients who have attended the Guy's Hospital Hypermobility Clinic over the past decade, many of whom have been observed over several years. A striking finding has been the number and variegated pattern of locomotor disorders suffered by individual patients. Many of the disorders encountered were amenable to treatment and serious disablement was seen in only a few individuals.

Case 1

Spondylolisthesis L4 root lesion

A 48-year-old male presented with a 1-year history of backache with radiation into the right buttock and anterior thigh. The pain had increased over the previous 3 months and was aggravated by sneezing. Examination revealed a markedly hypermobile spine (Fig. 7.1) with a step palpable at L4/5. The right femoral nerve stretch test was positive, the left being negative. Straight leg raising was 100° on both sides with negative sciatic nerve stretch tests. The right knee jerk was depressed, and there was sensory impairment over a patch below the right knee. A clinical diagnosis was made of a spondylolisthesis with right-sided L4 root lesion. Radiographs showed evidence of a grade 2 spondylolisthesis at L4/5 with narrowing of the disc space at this level and non-filling of the right L4 root sheath on radiculography (Figs. 7.2 and 7.3).

At operation the lamina of L4 was found to be totally mobile due to a bilateral defect in the pars interarticularis. The floating segment was excised and a moderate amount of fibrous tissue was noted at the site of the fracture. On both sides the L4 roots were tightly nipped between the prominent upper posterior corners of L5, the

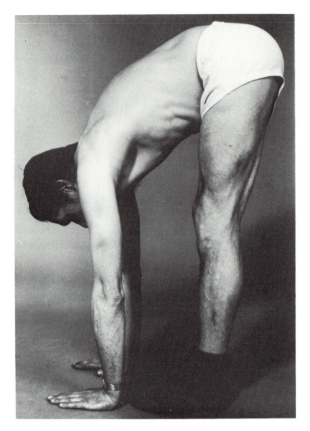

Fig. 7.1 Case 1. The patient demonstrating his ability to place the hands flat on the floor whilst bending forward with the knees straight. A 'step' is evident in the lumbar region.

pedicles of L4 and the site of the pseudoarthrosis. The roots were decompressed by removal of the surrounding fibrous tissue.

The patient was seen 4 months after the operation and was found to have some residual back pain and sciatica. The spine was mobile and the straight leg raise was not reduced.

Comment

This case illustrates how excessive mobility of the spine can be related to spondylolisthesis with resultant displacement which can impinge on the nerve roots, causing radicular symptoms. The condition is amenable to surgical intervention.

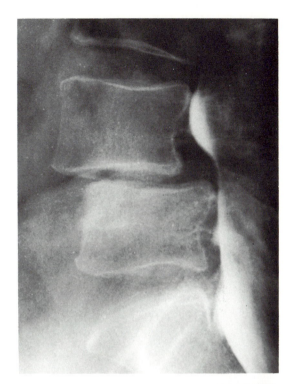

Fig. 7.2. Case 1. Radiculogram using metrisamide showing spondylolisthesis at L4/5.

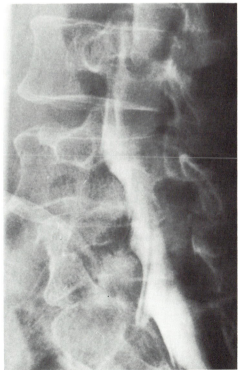

Fig. 7.3. Case 1. The L4 nerve root sheath on the right fails to fill.

Case 2

Ballet teacher with widespread osteoarthrosis affecting hands, left hip and left ankle

A female ballet teacher, aged 54 years, presented with a painful, swollen left ankle. She was found to be hypermobile with osteoarthrosis of the left ankle, left hip and small finger joints, with Heberden's and Bouchard's nodes. Treatment comprised physiotherapy and local steroid injection to the ankle. Surgery was considered but was not deemed to be indicated.

Comment

This patient had an hereditary predisposition to widespread osteoarthrosis (as evidenced by the Heberden and Bouchard's nodes). Whether the osteoarthrosis of the ankle and hip was attributable to her career as a ballet teacher is uncertain, though it may have been a contributory factor.

Case 3

Widespread osteoarthritis

Synovitis of MCP wrist and knee joints

Baker's cyst formation

Chondrocalcinosis

Cervical and lumbar spondylosis

Bilateral patellectomy

Left total hip replacement

Carpal tunnel syndrome

Misdiagnosis as rheumatoid arthritis

A 53-year-old female typist presented with polyarthritis of the metacarpophalangeal joints, wrists and knees of 6 months' duration. Initially she was thought to be suffering from rheumatoid arthritis. However she was persistently sero-negative with a normal ESR. Radiographically, degenerative changes were evident but erosions in her peripheral joints were not demonstrated.

The following year it was noted that she had widespread articular laxity (4/9 on the mobility scale) and the diagnosis was changed to the hypermobility syndrome. Her symptoms persisted, with recurrent synovitis of the knees and bilateral Baker's cyst formation, pain in the elbow, cervical and lumbar regions and swelling of the finger joints. In view of the persistent synovitis in association with subluxing patellae, bilateral patellectomy and partial synovectomy was performed (Fig. 7.4).

At operation it was observed that the femoral condyles and under-surfaces of the patellae were eburnated. Histologically there was hypertrophic villous synovitis. In spite of these procedures the synovitis persisted and

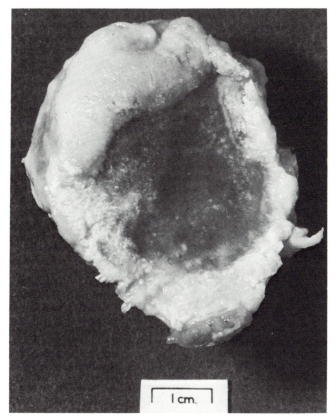

Fig. 7.4. Case 3. Patella removed at operation showing advanced osteoarthrotic changes over the femoral surface.

she became very depressed. At this point chondrocalcinosis was noted in her knee but not proven on microscopy of aspirated synovial fluid. The following year her left hip underwent a rapid deterioration and a total hip replacement was successfully carried out.

Comment

It is of interest that 10 years prior to her original presentation, she underwent bilateral median nerve decompression for carpal tunnel syndrome.

This case illustrates the rapidly progressive nature of the osteoarthrosis that may supervene in patients with generalised joint laxity, and how the diagnosis of the hypermobility syndrome may be missed.

Case 4

Recurrent synovitis of the knee with Baker's cyst formation

Ruptured Baker's cyst

Third degree Pott's fracture

Spontaneous fracture right calcaneum

Calcific tendonitis right shoulder

Back pain with left sciatica

'Disappearing disc'

Osteoarthrosis right knee with genu valgum

Varicose veins

Relief from acupuncture

A 52-year-old female hospital receptionist presented with pain in the left foot and on examination was found to have generalised hypermobility. Radiographs showed changes in the third and fourth left metatarsophalangeal joints which were suggestive of osteochondritis. The ESR was normal and the rheumatoid factor negative. Her condition responded to local steroid injections. Eight years previously she had suffered a Pott's fracture of the right ankle, which had been treated by internal fixation.

She subsequently developed varicose veins, recurrent synovitis of the right knee with effusion and Baker's cyst formation and an acute synovial rupture. Synovial fluid examination repeatedly revealed a viscous fluid with a very low cell count. Synovial biopsy demonstrated a mild, non-specific synovitis. The synovitis responded to an intra-articular steroid injection and rest.

She later presented with a 9-day history of right heel pain without obvious predisposing injury. Radiography revealed a fracture of the right calcaneum. Low back pain with left sciatic radiation then developed. Femoral and sciatic nerve stretch tests were positive, but there were no abnormal neurological signs. The episode settled with bed rest. Six months later the same symptoms recurred and persisted. Repeat radiography of the lumbar spine showed that the lumbo-sacral (L5-S1) disc had completely disappeared! (Fig. 7.5).

Additional clinic attendances were necessitated by acute supraspinatus tendonitis of the right shoulder and recurrent pain in the right knee. In addition to the synovitis of the right knee, a genu varum deformity developed in association with osteoarthritis of the medial compartment (Fig. 7.6).

Comment

In all, over a period of 7 years, the patient had made 27 outpatient attendances and had been in hospital three times because of her various locomotor problems. Following treatment with acupuncture and weight reduction, her attendance at the rheumatology clinic ceased and her symptoms are now minimal.

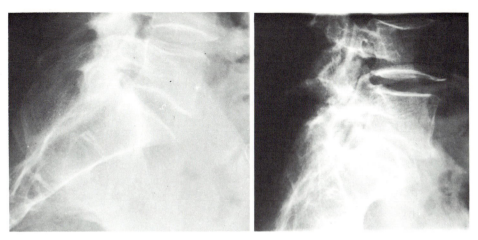

Fig. 7.5. Case 4. Sequential radiographs showing disappearance of the lumbosacral disc space occurring over a 6-month period.

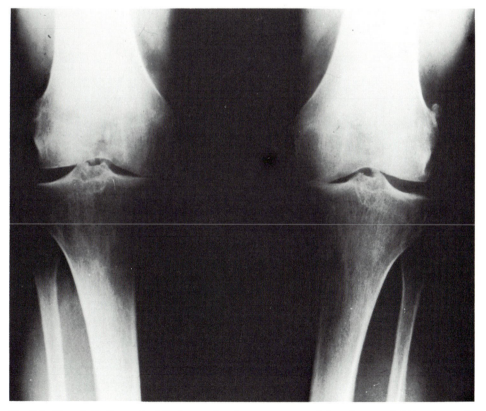

Fig. 7.6. Case 4. Radiograph of the knees showing genu varum deformity on weight bearing and osteoarthritis predominantly affecting the medial compartments.

Case 5

**Traumatic
synovitis PIP joint**

A 47-year-old woman fell from a train and suffered a hyperextension injury of her right middle finger. Examination revealed swelling of her third right proximal interphalangeal (PIP) joint with lack of full extension (Fig. 7.7). She had generalised hypermobility (6/9 on the mobility scale). Investigations, including a blood count, ESR, rheumatoid factor and radiographs were all normal. A diagnosis of traumatic synovitis was made and she responded to an intra-articular injection of methyl prednisolone.

Comment

Traumatic synovitis in a solitary joint is not uncommon in subjects with lax joints. It may, if untreated, become chronic. Response to intra-articular steroid injections is most satisfactory.

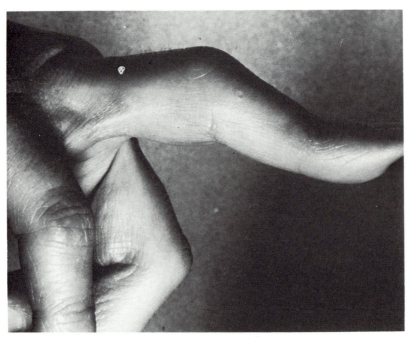

Fig. 7.7. Case 5. Synovitis of the PIP with fixed flexion deformity. The hyperextension of the MCP and DIP joints which is evident compensated for the loss of PIP joint movement.

Case 6

Cervical myelopathy due to large disc protrusion at C4/5 level with cord compression

Flexion deformity left thumb

Chronic synovitis left knee with Baker's cyst formation progressing to osteoarthrosis with valgum deformity

Supraspinatus tendonitis right shoulder

A 54-year-old woman presented with parasthaesiae in both arms and weakness of the left arm and leg. She also had a fixed flexion deformity of the interphalangeal joint of her left thumb. Examination revealed generalised hypermobility, a left-sided hemiparesis with sensory loss over the fourth left cervical dermatome and a loss of pain and vibration sensation over the right side of the body below the neck. Cord compression was confirmed by myelography (Fig. 7.8) and a cervical decompression and fusion resulted in a good recovery (Fig. 7.9). Shortly afterwards the interphalangeal joint of the right thumb was arthrodesed.

Over the ensuing 10 years her main problems have been a persistent synovitis of the left knee associated with a large popliteal cyst (Fig. 7.10). Repeated examination of synovial fluid revealed low cell counts and absence of crystals. Treatment was by intra-articular steroid injections and although synovectomy was considered at one

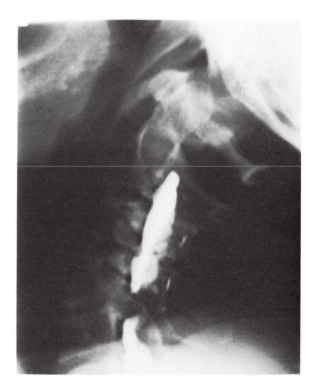

Fig. 7.8. Case 6. Pre-operative myelogram showing interruption of the column of Myodil due to a large cervical disc prolapse at C4/5.

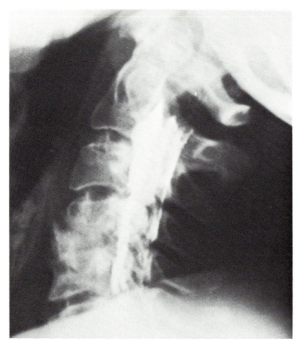

Fig. 7.9. Case 6. Post-operative myelogram showing anterior cervical fusion and restoration of the continuity of the contrast column.

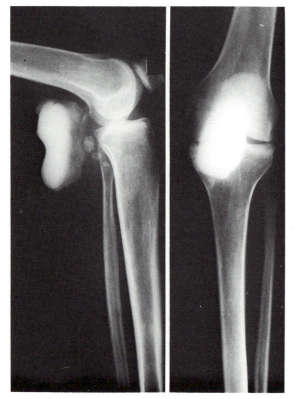

Fig. 7.10. Case 6. Popliteal cystogram delineating a large Baker's cyst in the left popliteal fossa.

stage, this was never undertaken. The Baker's cyst persisted and she gradually developed a left genu valgum deformity due to instability. The knee also became crepitant because of osteoarthrosis. Her only other rheumatological complaint was a single short-lived episode of supraspinatus tendonitis.

Comment

It is possible that laxity of the cervical spine was a pathogenic factor in this patient's cervical disc lesion, which resulted in cord compression. Fortunately, surgical intervention was completely successful. She also showed a gradually progressive osteoarthrosis of the knees accompanied by the formation of a Baker's cyst.

Case 7

Spontaneous dislocation of shoulder joints

A 16-year-old school girl complained of spontaneous dislocation of her shoulders when swimming backstroke. She was noted to have hypermobility of her hips and wrists. There were no other clinical abnormalities.

Comment

Treatment comprised reassurance of the patient, her parents and her physical education teachers concerning the benign nature of her condition.

Recurrent (and often spontaneous) dislocation of the joints was one of the important features of joint laxity described in the early literature.

Case 8

Dorsal root pain mimicking appendicitis

A 19-year-old girl presented with a 2-month history of pain in the right groin and iliac fossa and at operation a normal appendix was removed. She was later referred to the rheumatology clinic, where widespread hypermobility of the spine and peripheral joints (7/9 on the mobility scale) was noted. The right groin pain could be reproduced by left lateral flexion of the lumbar spine and a band of hyperaesthesia was found which conformed to the right D12 dermatome (Fig. 7.11).

There was no radiological abnormality to correspond with the presumed source of the D12 nerve root irritation, although a disc lesion at this level was the most likely explanation. She was referred to the physiotherapy department and 2 months later her pain had remitted.

Comment

This case illustrates how the origin of referred pain may be misconstrued and even lead to unnecessary surgery.

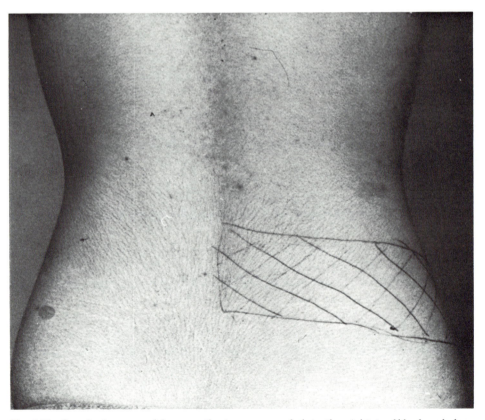

Fig. 7.11. Case 8. An area of hyperaesthesia corresponded to the right twelfth dorsal dermatome.

Case 9

Severe arthralgia since childhood

Intractable cervical dorsal and lumbar spinal pain

Symptomatic mitral valve prolapse

Mild bilateral sciatica

Carpal tunnel syndrome

Fractured pelvis

This 39-year-old woman presented with a 28-year history of severe joint and spinal pain precipitated by any strenuous activity. All athletic and sporting pursuits, both in her adolescence and in her adult life, had been severely curtailed. Her knees, hips, elbows, thumb bases and cervical, dorsal and lumbar spine were all affected.

She developed knee effusions after exercises whilst at school, but more recently signs of synovitis were absent. Treatment involving physiotherapy, osteopathy, analgesics, acupuncture and herbal remedies was uniformly fruitless and her principal relief came from rest. Her symptoms tended to improve during pregnancy and on at least one occasion worsened after giving birth. Routine blood investigations were negative and radiographs of the symptomatic areas were consistently normal. At the age of 18 she had fractured her pelvis after falling from a horse. When seen initially after the accident she had mild bilateral sciatica and bilateral carpal tunnel syndrome. Her mobility score was 7/9.

From the age of 39 she developed episodes of left inframammary chest pain associated with dizziness and breathlessness. Examination revealed a late systolic click and a murmur. An echocardiogram confirmed the presence of some degree of mitral valve prolapse. An ECG and a multiple gated isotope angiogram showed evidence of mild myocardial disease.

Comment

This patient now leads a very restricted life on account of her arthralgia. Her cardiac condition, by comparison, gives rise to few symptoms. The coincidence of arthralgia and widespread hypermobility together with mitral valve prolapse is suggestive of a generalised disorder of collagen in this patient.

Case 10

Bilateral patellectomy for osteochrondritis

Prolapsed intervertebral disc

Widespread arthralgia

Torn meniscus

Probable mitral valve prolapse

Supraspinatus tendonitis

A nursing sister in her late teens underwent bilateral patellectomy for severe osteochondritis. At the age of 19 she suffered an episode of lumbar disc prolapse with left-sided sciatica, which resolved with rest. The following year she complained of arthralgia of her hands, feet and knees with marked early morning stiffness. She was noted to have generalised laxity of her joints (5/9 on the mobility scale) and the hypermobility syndrome was diagnosed. Two years later she presented with a right-sided supraspinatus tendonitis and thereafter underwent a meniscectomy for a tear in a degenerate right-sided medical meniscus. An echocardiogram (taken as part of a survey) revealed probable mitral valve prolapse, which is symptom-free. She is now fit and well.

Comment

This case, like many of the others, illustrates the diverse nature of the symptoms which may be ascribed to joint laxity.

Case 11

Shallow acetabulae

Early osteoarthrosis

A 39-year-old woman gave a 9-year history of pain in both hips which was worse after physical activity. She had generalised hypermobility (6/9 on the mobility scale) and radiographs showed shallow acetabulae with loss of apical joint space and a tendency to subluxation of the hip. Her symptoms were not considered severe enough to warrant surgical intervention.

Comment

It seems likely here that the osteoarthrosis which developed in her dysplastic hips may have been promoted by the joint laxity.

Case 12

Cervical disc prolapse and spondylosis

Lumbar spine instability with severe spondylosis and spinal stenosis

Lumbar decompression on two occasions

Supraspinatus tendonitis

Osteoarthritis of hands, knees and shoulders

Chondrocalcinosis of knees

A 61-year-old male courier had suffered a cervical disc prolapse at the age of 36, with a recurrence of symptoms 8 years later. Both episodes were treated conservatively. At the age of 53 he underwent laminectomy for spinal stenosis associated with instability of L3/4/5. These abnormalities had given rise to cauda equina compression, complicated by a hypertrophic neuropathy. In turn, this had resulted in marked weakness in the left leg. The initial response to surgery was favourable but the symptoms recurred and a second operation was performed 6 years later. Other problems included widespread osteoarthritis of his hands, knees and shoulders with advanced cervical and lumbar spondylosis radiographically evident. Chondrocalcinosis was also present in his knees. His mobility score was 6/9.

Comment

This case illustrates the severe degenerative changes that may occur both in the cervical and in the lumbar spines of lax individuals, and the serious sequelae such as disc prolapse and spinal stenosis.

Case 13

Ballet dancer with bilateral medial ligament strain of knee

Chondromalacia patellae

An 18-year-old ballet student was unable to dance due to pain over the medial aspects of both knees. She showed generalised hypermobility (9/9) with marked bilateral genu recurvatum. The medial knee ligaments were tender bilaterally but responded to local steroid infiltration. A year later she presented with chrondromalacia patellae which resolved after treatment with short wave and exercises in the physiotherapy department.

Comment

Both ligamentous lesions and chondromalacia patellae are frequently seen in patients with lax knees, especially those who pursue vigorous exercise.

Case 14

Prolapsed intervertebral disc

A 59-year-old retired female dancer presented with a 6-week history of acute sciatica. She had an absent left ankle jerk and a left-sided sensory and motor deficit in the distribution of S1. Her mobility score was 7/9. Straight leg raising was reduced to 90° on the left with a positive sciatic nerve stretch test, compared with 120° on the right with a negative test. A radiculogram confirmed the presence of a prolapsed intervertebral disc with compression of the S1 nerve root on the left. She responded to an epidural steroid injection and made an uninterrupted recovery.

Comment

This case illustrates that in hypermobile subjects the normal straight leg raising test may be in excess of 100°, so that a reduction to 90° may be significant.

Case 15

Cervical and lumbar spondylosis

Shoulder capsulitis

Osteoarthritis thumb bases

Depressive state

A 47-year-old woman with generalised hypermobility had a 25-year history of back pain which was thought to be due to chronic disc prolapse. She also experienced pain due to cervical and dorsal spondylosis and was troubled with osteoarthritis of the first carpo-metacarpal joints and capsulitis of the right shoulder. She returned to hospital with the same symptoms on several occasions during the subsequent 7 years. During this period the clinical and radiological manifestations of osteoarthrosis progressed and she developed Heberden's and Bouchard's nodes. Her problems culminated in a depressive state which required psychiatric treatment.

Comment

It is not surprising that chronic pain arising from a number of identifiable lesions, as in this case, should lead to severe depression.

Case 16

Widespread arthralgia

Anxiety-depression

Mitral valve prolapse and regurgitation

Misdiagnosed as rheumatoid arthritis

A 54-year-old housewife experienced pains in her hands, wrists, elbows, left temporomandibular joint and cervical and lumbar spine during her late thirties. She was initially diagnosed as suffering from rheumatoid arthritis but this was never substantiated. She was formerly very athletic and able to perform contortionist manoeuvres, but after the onset of her symptoms she became stiff and immobile. Although she had lost much of her earlier joint laxity, her mobility score was 4/9. Her disability was complicated by a chronic depressive illness with phobic features. Radiographs showed mild widespread degenerative joint and spinal disease.

She was helped by non-steroidal anti-inflammatory drugs and hydrotherapy. Asymptomatic mitral regurgitation had been diagnosed at the age of 39 and this was later shown to be associated with mitral valve prolapse.

Comment

Her aortic compliance was exceptionally high, and this finding together with her mitral valve prolapse and joint laxity is suggestive of a widespread collagen disorder. Her daughter, mother and maternal aunt have suffered from similar articular problems.

Case 17

Widespread arthralgia

Carpal tunnel syndrome

Ulnar neuritis

Subluxation right inferior radio-ulnar joint

Colles' fracture

Osteoarthrosis of hands and knees

A middle-aged female potter with generalised hypermobility complained of aches and pains in various joints since her teens. Her shoulders, elbows, wrists, hands, knees and lower back were predominantly involved. In addition, she developed a right carpal tunnel syndrome (associated with subluxation of the right inferior radio-ulnar joint) which responded to local steroid injections. An episode of left ulnar neuritis was thought to be related to irritation of the nerve in the vicinity of the hypermobile elbow joint. While under observation she showed unequivocal evidence of generalised osteoarthrosis with Heberden's nodes and crepitus in both knees.

**Asymptomatic
mitral valve
prolapse**

Echocardiography undertaken as part of a survey showed marked mitral valve prolapse which was confirmed by the finding of a mitral click. Aortic compliance was also found to be abnormal.

Her joint symptoms were helped by non-steroidal anti-inflammatory drugs, but her carpal tunnel eventually required decompression. She sustained a Colles' fracture after minimal trauma.

Comment

As with the preceding case, the articular, mitral valve and bone problems in this woman were suggestive of a systemic collagen disorder.

Case 18

**Spondylolysis and
spondylolisthesis**

A 17-year-old girl presented with a history of low back pain since the age of 11. When 13 years of age, she commenced gymnastics and the pain became worse. At 15 years she began to experience painful locking of the

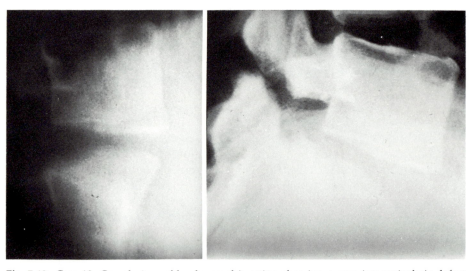

Fig. 7.12. Case 18. Coned view of lumbosacral junction showing a pars interarticularis defect with anterior slipping of L5 on S1 in extension (right-hand photograph) which is not seen in the flexed position (left-hand photograph).

back on bending forwards. These attacks would last for
up to 24 hours and occurred with increasing frequency. A
myelogram was normal. Although she was an active
healthy girl, she was precluded from normal sporting
activities.

Examination revealed widespread joint hypermobility
and radiographs showed a pars interarticularis defect
associated with an isthmic spondylolisthesis at L5/S1.
This was unstable with forward slip of L5 on S1 during
extension (Fig. 7.12). Spinal fusion was offered but de-
clined. When seen 10 months later her back was much
more comfortable and the instability which had been
evident on the earlier films was no. longer present
(Fig. 7.13). She was advised to avoid hyperextension
wherever possible and taught to practise isometric lumbar flexion exercises.

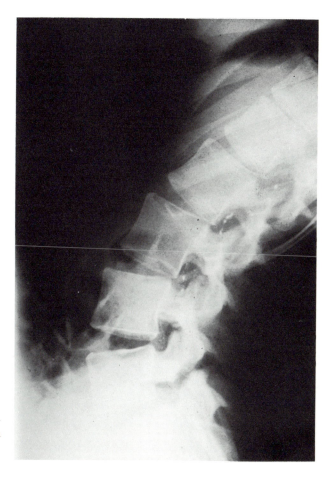

Fig. 7.13. Case 18. The earlier
instability on extension shown
in Fig. 7.12 is no longer
present.

Comment

Her skin was soft and stretchy and she was thought possibly to have a mild form of the Ehlers–Danlos syndrome.

Case 19

Premature osteoarthrosis: right hip

A 34-year-old model presented with a 5-month history of pain and stiffness in the left hip. This developed after she had moved to a new house with three flights of stairs to which she was not accustomed. Examination showed generalised hypermobility with reduction in hip joint movement, notably medial and lateral rotation. Radiographs revealed narrowing of the joint space superiorly with sclerosis of the acetabular aspect and flattening of the femoral head (Fig. 7.14). Her mobility score was 4/9.

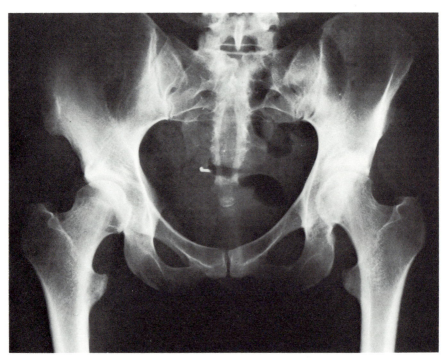

Fig. 7.14. Case 19. AP view of the pelvis. The left hip joint space is reduced, particularly in the superior region.

Comment

It is interesting that the patient's symptoms only developed when she was forced to undertake unaccustomed physical exercise.

Case 20

Flat feet

A 17-year-old ballet student complained of aching feet at the end of the day. Her teacher had noted 'fallen arches'. Examination showed bilateral pes planus and a mobility score of 9/9. Her symptoms responded to intrinsic foot exercises.

Comment

Flat feet are a common concomitant of joint laxity. Response to treatment is usually good.

Case 21

**Myotonia
congenita**

A 14-year-old girl presented with a 10-year history of stiffness and occasional pain in the muscles of her calves and thighs and in her finger joints and right knee. She found running and climbing stairs to be difficult on account of her muscle symptoms. There was no relevant family history.

Examination revealed widespread joint hypermobility (score 5/9) with marked myotonia in the muscles of all four limbs. An EMG confirmed the myotonia.

Comment

It was thought that the myotonia congenita was probably of the autosomal recessive variety and that the association with hypermobility was probably fortuitous. However, the concurrence of two hereditary disorders is of more than passing interest.

Case 22

Tenosynovitis of the wrist

A 15-year-old girl complained of a tender swelling over the dorsum of her left wrist and was found to have generalised joint laxity (mobility score 5/9). Her symptoms were relieved by the use of a splint, but they recurred from time to time especially after writing for prolonged periods.

Comment

The tenosynovitis was probably aggravated, if not initiated by her joint laxity.

Case 23

Chronic back strain in a male dancer

A 21-year-old male ballet dancer attended the clinic with recurrent low back pain. He had joint laxity, but no identifiable structural cause could be found on either clinical or radiological examination. He was referred to the physiotherapy department for muscle strengthening exercises and advised to abstain from dancing for 3 months. He was lost to follow-up.

Comment

The majority of acute episodes of acute back pain in dancers are probably due to ligamentous or muscle damage. Fortunately, they are self-limiting.

Case 24

Generalised osteoarthrosis

Recurrent dislocation of the left patella

A 42-year-old woman gave a 14-year history of pain in her knees, wrists and low back region which rendered her incapable of continuing her work as a dressmaker. She had previously dislocated her left patella on two occasions. Examination revealed Heberden's and Bouchard's

nodes, osteoarthrosis of her thumb base joints and knees
and some degenerative changes in the lumbar spine. She
had a mobility score of 7/9.

Comment

A number of similar patients have been seen over the
years with a combined picture of widespread joint laxity
and the nodal form of generalised osteoarthrosis. The
question arises as to whether this combination is anything
more than a chance association of two common hereditary disorders.

Case 25

Spondylolisthesis   A 63-year-old woman presented with a 6-month history
of pain in the left buttock which radiated to the knee and
was exacerbated by sneezing. She was obese and showed
a markedly hypermobile spine with a straight leg raise of
130° on both sides! Radiographs confirmed spondylolisthesis at L4/5 which appeared to be of the degenerative
(pseudo-spondylolisthesis) variety (Fig. 7.15). She was

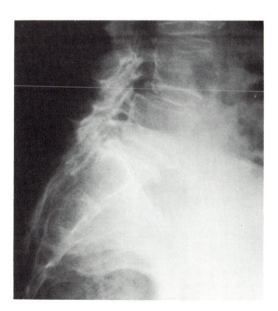

Fig. 7.15. Case 25. Lateral radiograph of
the lumbosacral junction showing
degenerative spondylolisthesis at L4/5.

helped by exercise therapy although she continued to complain of backache after strenuous activity.

Comment

This case is another example of spondylolisthesis in a hypermobile spine with nerve root compression causing sciatic pain.

Case 26

Widespread osteoarthrosis with spondylolisthesis and deformities of the forefeet

An obese hypermobile 68-year-old woman presented with pain in the shoulders, low back and feet. She was found to have Heberden's nodes and osteoarthritis in her knees, hands, ankles, tarsal and tarsometatarsal joints, together with hallux valgus. She was also noted to have a degenerative spondylolisthesis at L4/5. She was treated with anti-inflammatory drugs and weight reduction.

Comment

This patient has generalised osteoarthrosis of the hands and feet in association with a degenerative spondylolisthesis.

Case 27

Instability of the ankle in a ballet dancer

Chondromalacia patellae

Synovitis of toe joint

Ganglion

A 19-year-old ballet dancer presented with a 2-year history of 'giving way' of the right ankle which interfered with her dancing. She was found to be strikingly hypermobile (7/9 on the mobility scale). The right ankle showed evidence of instability. This was alleviated by increasing muscle tone through appropriate exercise.

The following year she reappeared with chondromalacia patellae in the left knee. Quadriceps exercises, avoiding hyperextension, and short wave diathermy produced considerable improvement. A year later she attended with traumatic synovitis of the first right metatarsopha-langeal joint. This was treated with ultrasound and settled within 2 months. Two years later she came to the clinic with a ganglion on the dorsum of the right big toe. She refused surgery.

Comment

This case history records 5 years of attendance at the ballet dancers' clinic at Guy's Hospital. It is fortunate that the patient's problems were minor and amenable to treatment.

Case 28

Osteoarthrosis of the knees and thumb base joints

A 57-year-old loose-jointed social worker developed pain-ful joints at the base of her thumbs at the age of 28 and over the next 20 years experienced gradually worsening pain in the knees. Her 27-year-old daughter was known to be hypermobile. Examination revealed marked osteo-arthrosis of the knees and thumb base joints and wide-spread hypermobility (5/9).

Comment

An unusual feature was the collapse of the right upper medial tibial plateau, which caused a genu varum de-formity and resulted in a bizarre gait. Operative replace-ment of the knee joint was considered but rejected.

Case 29

Arthralgia–influence of pregnancy

A 35-year-old hypermobile woman complained of arthral-gia of the elbows, hands, knees and toes which de-veloped during the course of her first pregnancy. The symptoms recurred during the first month of her second pregnancy, even before she realised that she was preg-nant, and became severe during the last trimester. She became symptom-free after the puerperium. In her third pregnancy, 2 years later, her activities were restricted owing to recurrent antepartum haemorrhage and she did not suffer from joint pains until 7 days after delivery.

She subsequently developed a synovitis of the right elbow after a fall. This problem and her other joint symptoms resolved spontaneously. After a further 18 months, polyarthralgia with early morning stiffness recurred in her right shoulder, interphalangeal joints, knees and toes. On this occasion she was not pregnant and her symptoms persisted for 2 years without evidence of synovitis. They were aggravated by extremes of hot or cold weather.

Comment

The exacerbation or arthralgia by pregnancy is unusual in the hypermobility syndrome and more often patients report amelioration of their symptoms.

Case 30

Osteoarthrosis of the knees

Baker's cyst formation

Pes planus

A 54-year-old obese lady gave a 2-year history of pain in both kness. Examination revealed generalised joint hypermobility with pes planus. She had bilateral valgus deformity of the knees with crepitus and lateral instability (Fig. 7.16). An effusion was present in the left knee and Baker's cysts were palpable in both popliteal fossae (Fig. 7.17). Radiographs showed degenerative changes in the knees with marked narrowing of the lateral compartments (Figs. 7.18 and 7.19). Contrast arthrography confirmed the presence of Baker's cysts.

Comment

This case is a good example of Baker's cyst formation in a patient with synovitis of the knees secondary to joint laxity.

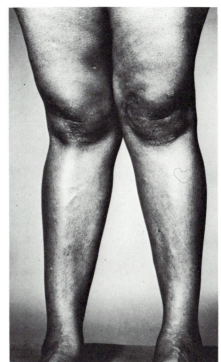

Fig. 7.16. Case 30. Valgum deformities of the knees during weight bearing.

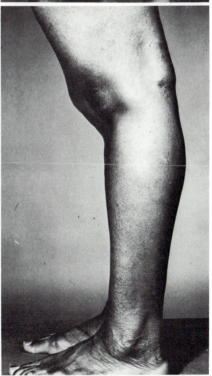

Fig. 7.17. Case 30. Marked genu recurvatum during weight bearing. A Baker's cyst is visible in the popliteal fossa.

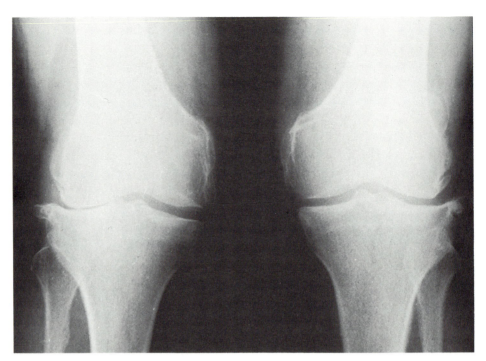

Fig. 7.18. Case 30. AP radiograph of the knees showing advanced osteoarthrosis predominantly affecting the lateral compartments, with a resulting valgum deformity.

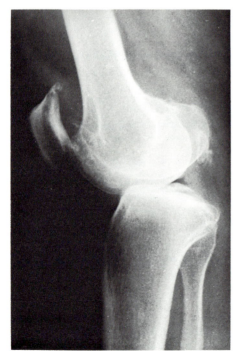

Fig. 7.19. Case 30. Lateral radiograph of the knee showing advanced osteoarthrosis of the patello-femoral and tibio-femoral compartments, with hyperextension on weight bearing.

Case 31

Various
misdiagnoses

Rheumatic fever

A 16-year-old girl was thought to have rheumatic fever at the age of six on the basis of pain and swelling of the elbows and right knee. Her joint pains recurred intermittently for periods of 6 to 9 months and she consulted numerous paediatricians and rheumatologists.

Examination at the age of 16 revealed mild synovitis of her wrists and elbows with effusions in both knees and tenderness over the joints of both great toes. She had widespread articular laxity with a score of 5/9 and the diagnosis was changed to the hypermobility syndrome. Her symptoms responded to restriction of exercise.

Comment

It is noteworthy that symptoms of hypermobility syndrome may be erroneously ascribed to other conditions.

Case 32

Synovitis of the
wrist joint

A 58-year-old woman complained of recurrent pain and swelling of the right wrist which started after pulling a heavy wardrobe, but recurred after other strenuous activities. She had a warm, swollen wrist with limited movement and hypermobility of the metacarpophalangeal thumb and wrist joints. Laboratory investigations yielded normal results and monoarthritis of the right wrist secondary to hypermobility was diagnosed. The synovitis resolved following the use of a splint.

Comment

The diagnostic clue in this case was the relationship of the onset of symptoms to trauma and the subsequent aggravation by physical activity. Trauma is the most important known pathogenetic factor in the development of articular symptoms in persons with joint laxity.

8. Hypermobility in the Performing Arts and Sport

Individuals endowed with hypermobility may excel in certain artistic occupations. The professional activities of ballet dancers, contortionists, musicians and sportsmen are all influenced by their range of joint movements. The wider implications of this situation are reviewed in this chapter.

Ballet Dancers

Are Ballet Dancers Born or Made?

In the performance of their art, ballet dancers display impressive ranges of joint movement which are clearly beyond the ability of lesser mortals. How much of this joint laxity is the result of painstaking regular training, often initiated in childhood, and how much is it due to an inherent laxity that may have acted in favour of recruitment to dancing? The answer is almost certainly that both factors are operative.

In order to test the hypothesis that generalised hypermobility may confer positive advantage in the selection of would-be ballet dancers for training, a comparative study of joint mobility was undertaken in 53 students attending the Royal Ballet School in London and 53 student nurses at Guy's Hospital (Grahame and Jenkins 1972). The results showed that compared with the nurses, the ballet students showed a significantly higher incidence of hypermobility of joints, not only of the spine, hips and ankles, which would be affected by training, but also of joints such as the knee, elbow and wrist which become unaesthetic in the hypermobile range (Fig. 8.1). Interestingly, 13% of the dancers but none of the nurses knew of a first-degree relative who suffered from recurrent knee effusions (a known complication of hypermobility), supporting the concept that generalised hypermobility can be inherited.

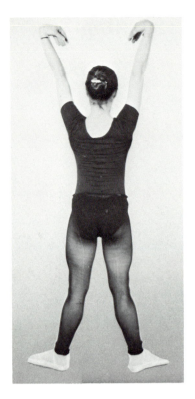

Fig. 8.1. Hyperflexion of the wrists and hyperextension of the elbows produces an unaesthetic appearance.

Is Generalised Joint Laxity an Asset or a Liability in Ballet Dancing?

On the credit side is the increased facility for undertaking the spectacular range of movement, notably of the spine, hips and ankles, that is required of a ballet dancer. In the tighter-jointed individual this can be achieved only by dint of hard work (if at all!).

On the debit side generalised laxity of ligaments can pose problems for the dancer. Indeed, an enhanced range of movement may result in an unacceptable appearance. This is seen, for example, in the so-called 'swayback knee' or genu recurvatum (Fig. 8.2). However, even when gross, this can be corrected satisfactorily by careful voluntary muscular control (Fig. 8.3). Hyperlaxity of the tarsal joints and the first tarso-metatarsal joint of the great toe (Fig. 8.4) can create serious and even disastrous problems when attempting to dance 'en pointe'. To a certain extent this lack of stability can be circumvented by improving muscular tone with exercise therapy.

Hypermobile dancers are vulnerable to all the ailments to which loose-jointed persons are susceptible, but because of the greater physical demands imposed by ballet dancing they are at even greater risk.

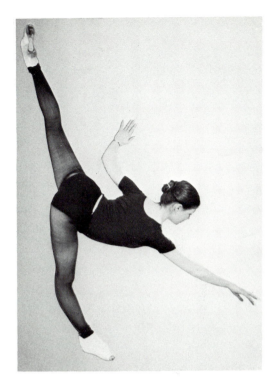

Fig. 8.2. The 'swayback knee'.

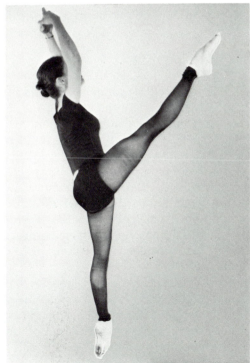

Fig. 8.3. The same knee corrected by
voluntary muscular control.

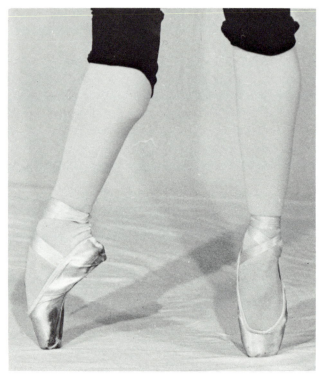

Fig. 8.4. Instability of the first metatarsophalangeal joint precludes the possibility of dancing 'en pointe'.

Miller et al. (1974) compared the problems of the professional ballet dancer with those of a vigorous athlete, and cited osteochondral fractures, fatigue fractures, sprains, chronic ligamentous laxity of the knee, meniscal tears, degenerative arthritis of multiple joints and low back pain as problems which were frequently encountered.

In a systematic radiological survey of 28 members of the Cincinatti Ballet Company evidence of stress fractures was seen in the weight-bearing bones of the lower limbs (Schneider et al. 1974). These were recognised in the femoral necks, anterior aspects of the mid-shafts of the tibiae and the lower half of the fibulae. In the feet, cortical thickening was present in the first, second or third metatarsal shafts in 23 out of 28 dancers but there were no fractures.

A postal survey of injuries sustained in dancing, conducted throughout the United States and some other countries, revealed that ligamentous injuries were by far the commonest lesions (Washington 1978). These occurred in the knee, ankle and foot, in descending order of frequency. Fractures constituted the second most frequent injury and the majority of these were in the metatarsals and phalanges.

Scintigraphy has been used to bring to light stress lesions in dancers presenting with pain and tenderness in the bones of the foot with normal appearance on radiography (Grahame et al. 1979). Such a case is illustrated in Figs. 8.5 and 8.6, when little is shown on conventional radiography although there is increased uptake in the scan in an area corresponding to the shaft of the second right metatarsal. This 16-year-old ballet student had experienced pain in the affected region for the previous 18 months and had been precluded from doing her point work. After a 3-month rest her symptoms remitted and a repeat bone scan was normal. Similar findings have been reported in athletes (El Sayed et al. 1979). If generalised joint laxity represents one aspect of a multisystem heritable connective tissue disorder, it is conceivable that fractures, at least in some dancers, may be a further facet of the same problem.

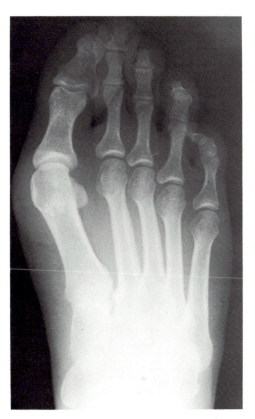 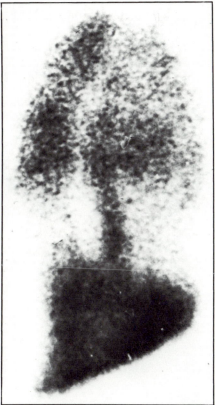

Fig. 8.5. Radiograph of the foot of a ballet dancer complaining of pain in the second right metatarsal shaft. There is hypertrophy of the cortex but no fracture.

Fig. 8.6. A scintiscan using technetium-99m diphosphonate. Increased uptake of the isotope in the region of the second right metatarsal is indicative of a 'stress lesion'.

Reproduced by kind permission of the editor and publishers of *Rheumatology and Rehabilitation*.

As many of the case histories cited in an earlier chapter testify, ballet dancers figure highly amongst the casualties of hypermobility and the variety of problems presenting in a ballet dancers' clinic is wide (Burry and Grahame 1973). Although the majority of lesions may be attributed to the effects of trauma and/or overuse, the vexed question as to whether dancing on hypermobile joints predisposes to premature osteoarthrosis remains unresolved.

It is interesting to note that in the Soviet Union, by contrast with the practice in the Western world, hypermobility is virtually an exclusion factor in the selection of ballet dancers (S. Marr, personal communication). Doubtless this is because of the high morbidity which occurs amongst lax-jointed dancers. In the Kirov Ballet, for example, only those children who show sufficient stability to enable standing on one foot in a supinated cavus position are selected for further training. Furthermore, the Russians seem to go en pointe from the mid-tarsal joints rather than from the first metatarsophalangeal joint, as is customary in western practice.

Ballet dancers combine an inherent tendency to articular hypermobility with life-long physical demands (Fig. 8.7). The study of their locomotor system is likely to yield dividends in terms of our knowledge of the natural history of joint laxity.

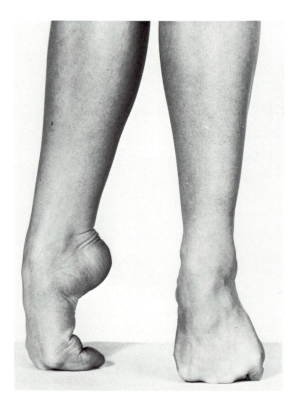

Fig. 8.7. The 'en pointé position places enormous long term mechanical stress on the musculo-skeletal structures of the feet.

Contortionists

Historical Background

Contortionists were certainly active 4000 years ago, as evidenced by an engraving on the hilt of the sword, which now rests in a museum at Heraklion, on the island of Crete. This depicts a lithe youth in the Palace of Knossos, balancing himself on the tips of his toes and the crown of his head, while arched over the point of the blade. Extreme joint laxity seems to have excited interest in many cultures; a figurine of an Inca contortionist is shown on the cover.

During medieval times, contortionists performed in fairgrounds, attracting an audience by their peculiar abilities. When a crowd gathered, their assistants would sell patent remedies, such as 'slippery worm oil', claiming that it was efficacious in the treatment of sore and stiff joints. The contortionist's performance was obvious proof of the benefits to be obtained from regular applications of the oil! These acts were the forerunners of America's 19th century travelling medicine show wagons.

Nosology and Semantics

There has been much confusion in the past as to the differences, from a professional point of view, between the 'India Rubber Man' and the 'Elastic Lady'. Although these terms were more or less interchangeable in the circus world, the India Rubber Man was usually a joint-bending contortionist, while the Elastic Lady was a skin-stretching exhibitionist. The elastic people could take hold of the skin of their face or trunk and pull it out for several inches. On release, it would immediately spring back into its former position. These individuals had the Ehlers–Danlos syndrome (EDS), which is a familial disorder of connective tissue (see Chap. 9). Articular hypermobility is also a feature of EDS and the elastic people were therefore equipped to perform contortions. However, in view of their cutaneous fragility and unstable joints, it is doubtful if they indulged in this activity.

The contortionist's act is centered around the ability to hyperextend or hyperflex the spine. In circus terminology, the performer is either a 'front bender' or 'back bender', and all the facets of the act are built on these movements. Many contortionists have considerable athletic prowess, and they may be able in indulge in such variations as placing their feet around their necks, while standing on one hand.

The forward bender is usually the 'funny man' as he can take up ludicrous positions and perform amusing feats. In contrast, the backward bender or 'posturer' has a more serious act. The posturer is often an attractive young woman who can perform speciality acts, or incorporate her abilities into a graceful dance routine.

Training

Many contortionists develop their skills by rigorous training. This must begin in childhood, and the French author, Guy de Maupassant, described how mountebanks would steal children for this purpose. Legislation to prevent training of children was enacted at the beginning of the present century, but the law is still permissive on the continent of Europe.

Contortionists who have acquired their joint laxity by years of training must practice for several hours each day, and even a week of inactivity will result in a marked stiffening of the joints. In the same way, a long warming-up period is required before the performance. However, some contortionists have inherent articular laxity, and these individuals are in a much more fortunate situation, as they require very little in the way of training or warming up. They are usually able to perform forward and backward bending with equal facility, and inactivity does not lead to loss of joint mobility (Figs. 8.8, 8.9 and 8.10). On the other hand, their joints may be unstable, and they may be unable to perform feats of strength. Although able to roll up into a tiny ball, they cannot do this while balanced on their fingers! This type of joint laxity is often a genetic trait, and these individuals may have familial undifferentiated hypermobility (see Chap. 10). The disorder is usually inherited as an autosomal dominant, and a number of affected persons are members of well-known circus families.

Socio-medical Implications

It is a surprising fact that osteoarthritis does not seem to affect elderly contortionists, and indeed, many of them retain hypermobility in old age. Ferry the Frog could still wrap his feet around his head at the age of 72, and he attributed his good health to his professional activity. Dad Witlock was performing in an American circus when he was 79 years old, and Norwood, the Flexible Fellow, retained much of his flexibility in his eighties (Fig. 8.11).

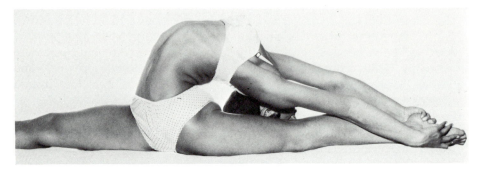

Fig. 8.8. A professional contortionist demonstrating her prowess. From Beighton (1970)

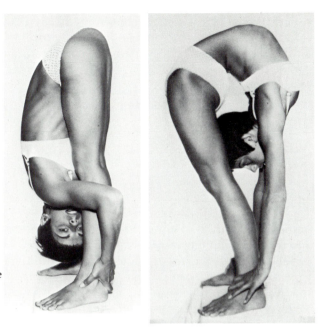

Fig. 8.9. and Fig. 8.10.
Contortionist with inherent
articular laxity are usually able
to perform forward and
backward bending with equal
facility. From Beighton (1970).

Fig. 8.9.   **Fig. 8.10.**

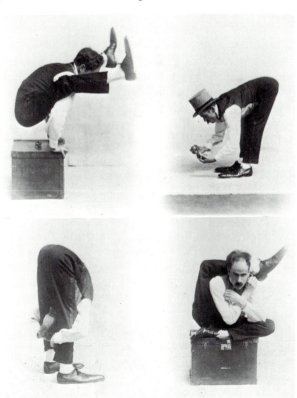

Fig. 8.11. 'Norwood the
Flexible Fellow', a professional
contortionist in the days of the
music halls.

Perhaps the secret of their continuing health is their good nature and their readiness to please other people. In the theatrical world it is axiomatic that the Elastic Ladies are always prepared to stretch a point, while the India Rubber people are renowned for their willingness to bend over backwards to be of assistance!

Musicians

Introduction

Manual dexterity is essential to the handling of many orchestral instruments and in these circumstances hypermobility may be an asset. The study of certain instrumentalists provides an opportunity for separating the acquired from the hereditary components of hypermobility. Dancers and contortionists tend to use both halves of the body equally. By contrast, musicians, such as string players, will perform quite different functions with their two hands. As such, they act as their own controls and this adds to the interest of studying this particular group.

The musician most frequently quoted as having extreme hand hyperlaxity is the Italian violinist and composer Niccolo Paganini (1782–1840). Born into a poor family, he had little opportunity for formal education. Several contemporary accounts describe his tall, thin frame and spider-like features. He apparently had a chest deformity and striking laxity of his hands. Indeed, it was this hand laxity that enabled him to compose works that could be played by few other violinists at the time, mainly because of the technical difficulties involved. It is uncertain whether he had simple familial hyperlaxity or whether, as seems more likely, he had an inheritable disorder of connective tissue such as the Marfan or Ehlers–Danlos syndrome.

The Hands in Instrumentalists

Individuals may find themselves particularly suited to certain instruments for a variety of reasons. For example, a person with perfect appreciation of pitch may use this to advantage by selecting a stringed instrument; those with less accurate pitch may be better suited to keyboard instruments. In the same way the anatomical structure of the hands relates to the many instruments which are available.

The modern fingering systems for woodwind instruments, such as the Boehm system for the clarinet, ensure that during performance both hands behave equally. Although it may be imagined that a small hand would be suited to the flute while a large hand would be appropriate for the bassoon, in practice the large number of keys provided on the modern bassoon mean that this instrument can be played with a fairly small hand. In the case of brass instruments the functions allotted to the two hands differ. However, modern valves and their positions ensure that the technical ability required of either hand in terms of stretching is not particularly great. Comparable use of both hands is made in playing keyboard instruments, but here, in view of the size of modern keyboards such as those on the piano, there may be greater opportunities for hands with wide span.

It is with stringed instruments, however, that the greatest disparity in hand function is found. The right hand is relegated to the relatively easy job of holding the bow. By contrast, the left hand not only spans the fingerboard to provide the correct string length, but also imparts a vibrato to the tone by the combination of impulses involving the muscles of the hand, wrist and arm. This effectively provides a continuous, almost imperceptible oscillation in the pitch of the notes. On the basis that prior to learning a string instrument both hands have equal ability, comparison of both hand function and disease in advanced string players allows enumeration of those problems that must have arisen by stretching of the (left) fingerboard hand and which, if absent on the right side, could not have been inherited. This form of analysis is of particular value in the study of classical guitarists and other string players.

Pianists

The instrument conventionally described as a pianoforte has evolved over the years. Not only have there been alterations in tone and improvements in mechanical efficiency, but the size of both keys and keyboards has altered. Comparison of the modern piano with that played by Mozart, for example, show that the earlier keyboard was much more compact. The increase in the size of the instrument, and therefore in the number of octaves spanned, occurred mainly during Beethoven's lifetime (1770–1827). Appraisal of the three main groups into which his piano sonatas can be divided clearly shows how the instrument became larger during this time. Only his last five piano sonatas are written for a piano of the seven and one third octave range that is familiar to us today.

These technical differences in the pianos over the centuries have to be taken into account in a historical survey. Nevertheless, it is possible to speculate on the hand capabilities of the different composers who also performed their own works from a study of the music that they produced. Thus, the music of Mozart is suited to small hands and involves a lot of delicate fingerwork to play the runs. Allowing for the style forced upon him, it seems that Mozart's hands could not have been particularly large and that it would not have been advantageous for him to be hypermobile. Beethoven's piano music, like that of Schumann, falls easily and conveniently under hands of normal size and of normal laxity.

During the romantic era there was a blossoming of virtuosity, but even allowing for this, different styles emerged. The piano music of Tschaikovsky for example, relies heavily upon the ability of the performer to span consecutive octaves, but does not often fully employ the middle fingers of the hands in chord work. In contrast, Brahms might have had hands of comparable span, but with relatively more lateral flexibility of the middle fingers in order to play the chords which are frequently found in his music.

Both Liszt and Rachmaninov are likely to have had considerable span as well as possessing significant articular laxity in the hands in order to play the difficult music which they wrote.

Although retrospective analysis may seem slightly fanciful, there is some justification. Plaster of Paris casts of Liszt's hand do exist and indeed show the hands to be relatively large. Pupils of Rachmaninov are still alive and their accounts leave no doubt that he had considerable lateral laxity of the middle fingers of the hands as well as a wide, spidery span. This enabled him to play with great ease the stretched chords that he so frequently composed.

It is uncertain whether these accomplishments were inherited or whether they arose by regular and strenuous practice. However, distinction must be made between the needs to practise to stretch hands and to strengthen muscles or to 'warm up' in order to reduce the 'gelling' stiffness of the hands that can quickly occur with disuse. Whether pianists with hyperlax hands are less susceptible than others to 'gelling' stiffness has never been adequately determined.

String Players

The attributes of Paganini have already been described. The violin, by virtue both of its size and tone, is better suited to pyrotechnics than the more cumbersome double bass or even the cello, and it is likely that individuals with hyperlax hands might particularly gravitate towards this instrument. However, the fingerboard of the violin is smaller than that of the cello, double bass or guitar and it is with these three instruments that a greater span and increased lateral laxity of the metacarpophalangeal joints might be advantageous. Once the span is achieved, the player is required to provide a vibrato tone, and this is perhaps most marked in the case of the guitar. Guitar playing, therefore, stretches the left hand to the utmost whilst requiring considerable muscular power and neuromuscular co-ordination to produce a tremulous effect with the hand held in the stretched position.

Comparison of the two hands in string players has several important scientific applications. In the first place, assuming both hands start with equal laxity, the effect of training on the stretched hand can be compared to the non-stretched hand. This is likely to be an amalgam not only of ligamentous suppleness, but also of muscle tone. Secondly, injuries that are suspected to be the result of joint hyperlaxity can be reliably ascribed to this factor if they are present only in the stretched left hand. Thirdly, study of patients suffering from the arthritides who subsequently go on to play instruments to an advanced level allows separation of the effect of stretching from that of pure mechanical trauma upon the natural history of the acquired rheumatic disease.

Clinical Aspects

The professional musician is often neglected by the medical profession. Athletes may have a coach, physiotherapist and a sports medicine clinic to attend to their acute and chronic injuries. Members of dancing companies also are likely to have access to a trained physiotherapist and an orthopaedic surgeon if they suffer injury.

In contrast, orchestras make no such arrangements for their players. Musicians have a schedule which is every bit as taxing as that of professional sportspeople or dancers and, more importantly, they enjoy a longer professional life. Futhermore, they have to keep their hand joints in perfect fitness throughout their career. Despite their obvious needs, little medical advice is ever supplied to musicians on the care of their hands. When consulted by musicians, rheumatologists are often in a position to treat minor abnormalities of the joints of the hands that might be ignored in an average person but which are incapacitating for a professional instrumentalist.

Musicians attending the Rheumatology Clinic at Leeds General Infirmary fall into three main categories: (a) those with hyperlaxity of the hands; (b) those with normal laxity of the hands but with overuse syndromes; (c) those who have acquired systemic rheumatic diseases but who still wish to continue their career. Case histories are presented from each of these three groups, with particular attention being paid to hypermobility.

Hyperlaxity: Traumatic Synovitis in a Classical Guitarist

P.D., a 31-year-old male, was a student of the classical guitar. He had practised for up to 5 hours each day for the last 10 years and was an advanced performer with a national reputation. In June 1978 he noticed pain at the back of the left wrist associated with swelling, exacerbated by practising the guitar. It was not present in the other hand and no other joints were involved. In December 1978 he sought the advice of his general practitioner and a cystic swelling on the dorsum of the left wrist was ascribed to traumatic synovitis (Fig. 8.12). He considered himself to be 'double-jointed' in comparison with other members of the class and there was an unusual degree of joint laxity present in both hands (Fig. 8.13). In May 1979 he was seen in the Rheumatology Clinic at Leeds General Infirmary. The swelling of the dorsal aspect of the left wrist had persisted, but his symptoms were controlled by indomethacin 25 mg tds. There was no early morning stiffness and no other symptoms apart from possible intermittent swelling of some proximal interphalangeal joints.

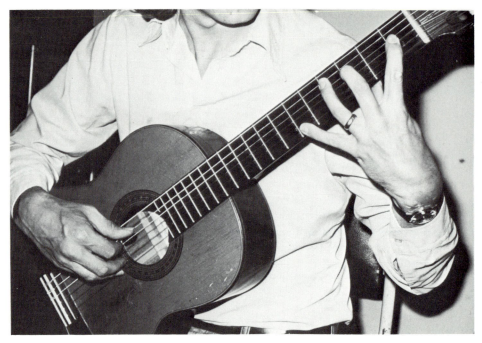

Fig. 8.12. The left wrist of the guitarist exhibiting untreated traumatic synovitis. From Bird and Wright (1981).

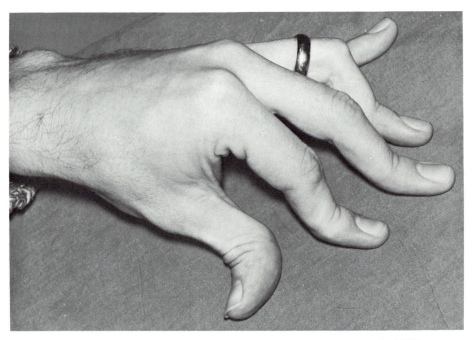

Fig. 8.13. The joints of the guitarist's hands were very lax. From Bird and Wright (1981).

His father had regarded himself as 'doubled-jointed' and a maternal aunt and grandmother were both said to have had rheumatoid arthritis.

Although his score for generalised hypermobility was only 4/9, he had marked hyperlaxity in both hands. There was no clinical evidence of rheumatoid disease at the metacarpal or metatarsal heads or at the ulna styloid. All other joints were normal.

Routine haematological and serological investigations yielded normal results and radiographs of the hands and feet revealed no abnormality.

He was treated with a single local injection of 2 mg triamcinolone hexacetonide and a short period of rest. This produced immediate and lasting improvement in spite of a subsequent return to regular guitar practice. He has had only minimal symptoms over the last 2.5 years; these have not required further steroid injection and are controlled by indomethacin capsules which are taken as required, 2 or 3 before a concert (Fig. 8.14).

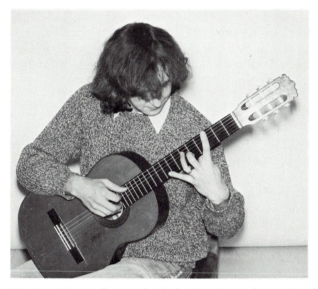

Fig. 8.14. The swelling resolved after injection with steriod and he was able to return to regular guitar practice. From Bird and Wright (1981)

The apparent association between the patient's joint laxity, his occupation and the synovitis prompted study of the other members of the guitar class (Bird and Wright 1981). Details were collected of age, sex and duration of guitar playing. Hyperextension of the metacarpophalangeal joint of the left index finger was measured by the Leeds finger hyperextensometer (Jobbins et al. 1979) and assessment of lateral laxity of the fingers made by eye and graded as +/++/+++. The finger hyperextensometer was also used to assess laxity of the same joint in 100 normal people, drawn at random from a Caucasian population.

The degree of joint laxity found in the other members of the guitar class (11 male; 3 female) was in no instance as marked as in this particular individual. Overall, the females exhibited slightly more laxity than the males. Hand laxity did not correlate with the duration of guitar playing, and the observations suggested that hereditary factors were more important than regular training in producing the observed laxity. Even when an allowance was made for the age differences, the only member of the class (P.D.) who exhibited synovitis had by far the most striking laxity in the hands. This was not only in an antero-posterior plane, but also in a lateral plane. Indeed, P.D. was the only member of the class who could reasonably be described as 'double-jointed'.

It is of interest that guitar players overall have a lower degree of hyperextension than normal members of the population. This possibly reflects their greater muscular control, since studies on athletes confirm that the range of movement at other joints in the body is reduced by regular athletic training (vide infra). In the case of P.D. there was a strong history of joint hyperlaxity on his father's side of the family and it seems his hyperlaxity was inherited. Only the stretched hand developed a synovitis and it is in this hand that he has had the majority of musculoskeletal symptoms associated with benign hyperlaxity. Lateral instability in the loaded joint may be the most important factor in the aetiology of traumatic synovitis.

Overuse Syndromes: Synovial Trauma in a Violinist

P.M. was a 27-year-old violinist, recently appointed as sub-leader of an orchestra of national acclaim. He had performed to a high standard for almost 10 years and played regularly in the evenings with the orchestra, rehearsing throughout the day. His symptoms had always been confined to the left hand and wrist and he had never had problems in the right hand. He attributed this fact to the greater stress placed upon this hand in his profession. By contrast to the previous patient, he did not consider himself to be double-jointed, and there was no evidence of generalised hypermobility.

He presented to the Leeds Rheumatology Clinic with a history of 4 weeks' pain at the left wrist. The pain was most pronounced on flexing this joint to an extreme degree and rapid fingerwork produced considerable discomfort. It subsided over a 24-h period when his work schedule allowed him to rest. In the past, there had been no swelling of the wrist or any other joint in either hand and there was no family history of arthritis.

Examination showed neither synovitis nor effusion in any of the joints of the left wrist or hand. The tendons were intact and moving well. There was no tethering and no pain in any tendon when the muscle attached to that tendon was worked against a resistance. There was, however, a localised point at which pain could be elicited on the extensor tendon expansion over the left wrist. This pain was most marked when the wrist was placed in a position of extreme flexion. Routine haematological and laboratory studies were within normal limits.

The most likely diagnosis appeared to be an overuse tear of the synovium or extensor tendon sheath which was slow to heal because of the constant movement at this site due to the performer's profession. The patient was subsequently able to completely immobilise the joint for 4 days and the symptoms disappeared. His schedule was then changed to a compromise between immobilisation and careful playing (without stretching of the joint) and the pain resolved over a period of 3 months.

The interest of this case is that it is in many ways reminiscent of the previous patient (P.D.), with the exception that this patient had no hyperlaxity. It seems that when hyperlaxity is present the instability causes a traumatic synovitis at the wrist joint with corresponding synovial hypertrophy. By contrast, with normal laxity, the soft tissues are more likely to respond to this situation by tearing. The fact that P.M.'s symptoms were localised to one hand strongly suggests that the mechanical aetiology was related to his playing. Comparable overuse syndromes causing non-specific pain, tendonitis (which resolves with local steroid injection) or synovial tears (as in this example) have been seen in other musicians including a flautist, a cellist and a pianist.

Acquired Systemic Disease: Generalised Osteoarthrosis in a Violinist

Mrs E.M., aged 68, first attended Leeds General Infirmary in October 1980. For almost 20 years she had been the leader (concert master) of a respected local orchestra. She had played the violin regularly for over 50 years and also taught this instrument. Her symptoms were in both hands and radiographs obtained at a 13-year interval showed progressive osteoarthrosis (Figs. 8.15 and 8.16). She also had degenerative changes in the cervical spine.

Examination confirmed the diagnosis of osteoarthrosis with the presence of Heberden's nodes and typical osteoarthritic deformity. There was no evidence of rheumatoid disease in the form of muscle wasting, vasculitis or synovial proliferation. The result of haematological and immunological investigations were normal and there was no radiological evidence of osteopenia or bony erosions.

It is noteworthy that this patient, according to her own history, which was presumed to be reliable, initially had joints which were of normal laxity. As the hand became progressively deformed she had acquired a number of tricks in order to cope with double stopping and arpeggios. This had caused her to develop, by training, a degree of hyperlaxity in the hand which she had not hitherto enjoyed. With this hypermobility she was able to play violin concertos and solo violin parts of quite considerable difficulty in her role as orchestral leader. To some extent her acquired laxity may have been due to earlier treatment with a small dose of prednisolone (2 mg per day) in an attempt to alleviate the joint symptoms. It was also of interest that serial radiographs taken over a period of almost 15 years showed a differential distribution of osteoarthrosis between the two hands. In the right hand, which held the bow, there had been striking radiological changes at the thumb base, perhaps because of the constant use required at this joint. By

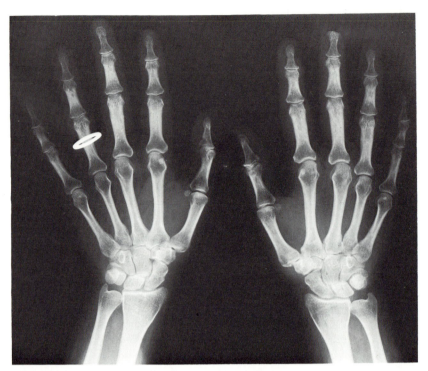

△ **Fig. 8.15.**   ▽ **Fig. 8.16.**

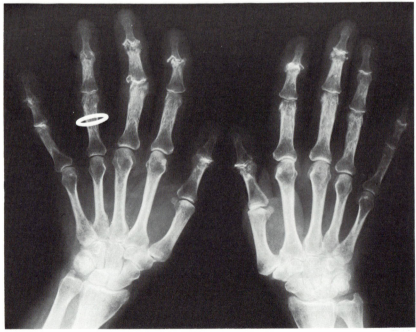

Fig. 8.15. and Fig. 8.16. Radiographs of the hands of a violinist taken at a 13-year interval. They demonstrate the development of osteoarthrosis at the joints under a strain, as detailed in the text.

contrast, in the left hand, the changes were predominantly at the distal interphalangeal joints, which were particularly involved in playing the strings. In the opposite hand these interphalangeal joints were almost spared. Clinically there was no evidence of hyperlaxity at other joints, apart from those in the left hand. She had been managed on a regular dose of a non-steroidal anti-inflammatory agent which was doubled or trebled on the day of an important concert. A cautious weaning off prednisolone has also been attempted, so far without success.

Musicians tend to be people of above average intelligence who, because of the close attention they pay to the joints in their hands, give a full and valuable history. Joint problems in musicians, whether or not they have hypermobility, is a field that has not hitherto received a great deal of attention from rheumatologists.

Sport

All sportspeople attest to the need for 'flexibility', a useful attribute which is said by coaches to improve performance in a wide variety of sports. There is a Gaussian distribution of 'flexibility' throughout the population and in sports this natural variation may be altered by regular training. A stiff person may become more supple but may never reach the level achieved by individuals who have greater natural endowment.

The range of movement at any given joint depends upon a variety of factors, including muscular tone, laxity of the ligaments and joint capsules and the shape of bony contours. In the hip, for example, either acetabular dysplasia or ligamentous laxity may produce an abnormally wide range of movement. Individuals must be considered on their own merits according to their sport, and different joints within the same person are likely to respond to different training programmes. For example all the best hurdlers may have a small degree of acetabular dysplasia which enables them to achieve the wide range of lateral movement at the hip joint that is required in this sport. Regular training of the individual without this particular bone structure may never achieve the range of movement required, no matter how much attention is given to the factors which may be altered, such as muscle tone and ligamentous stretching.

In Eastern European countries the selection of individuals who are suitable for particular sports has reached a high level of sophistication. Schoolchildren are screened for their body attributes and directed into the sport in which they are most likely to succeed. This selection is followed by a lengthy and detailed training programme at specialist state subsidised schools.

The range of movement that can be achieved at joints varies not only between persons but between different joints in the same individual. 'Flexibility' may not always be of value to the sportsperson. Joint hyperlaxity at the elbows, a feature deliberately sought on the Carter and Wilkinson scoring system, may be a severe disadvantage to a gymnast who has to stand on his or her hands. The elbows may give way under the weight of the body and regular training is required to increase the muscle tone around the elbow joint in order to achieve stabilisation. Similarly, hyperextension of the knee joint, a feature also sought in the Carter and Wilkinson scoring system, places runners at a disadvantage, particularly when running downhill. Conversely, the ability to hyperextend the knee confers a mechanical advantage in uphill running.

The virtue of evaluating joint laxity in sport is to enable the direction of each individual to the sport for which their joints are most suited. Thereafter, where necessary, training programmes should be directed at improving the performance of the joints in terms of the requirements of the particular sport. This may involve either inducing hyperlaxity in a stiff person or stabilising laxity in an individual who is initially too supple. Certain sports where hypermobility is especially relevant, or to which the author's attention has been directed, are reviewed below.

Gymnastics

In gymnastics hyperlaxity at numerous joints is of considerable advantage. Indeed the sport has much in common with ballet, which has already been discussed elsewhere in this chapter. A wide range of movement of the lumbar spine, particularly flexion and hyperextension, the hips and the shoulders is a pre-requisite and laxity is also required in the wrists, fingers and feet. The most extensive movements in the different set pieces are allocated to joints of ball and socket structure (the hip and the shoulder) or to joints that move synchronously, as do the intervertebral joints in the lumbar spine. By contrast, relative stability is useful at the elbows and the knees.

Women's gymnastics place great emphasis on suppleness at many joints. Men's gymnastics differ in that muscular power and the maintenance of balance are more important. In sports acrobatics strength and suppleness are combined in both men and women. Strength is required as the participants balance on each other's shoulders to build pyramids, and although the peak age of performance for the types of gymnastics which require suppleness is in the mid-teens, it is half a decade later in this latter sport.

Coaches in gymnastics prefer a relatively stiff newcomer to a novice who is too supple. It is easier to stretch joints either by active or passive exercise and thus confer acquired hyperlaxity, even though this may be lost in the absence of regular training, than to stabilise joints, such as the elbow, which are weakly muscled.

A routine gymnastic position such as the 'crab' (Fig. 8.17) can be achieved in a variety of ways. This posture is reached by summating a total of 180° of hyperextension so that both the feet and hands are on the floor, although the actual joints that are used may vary according to the individual. A few will

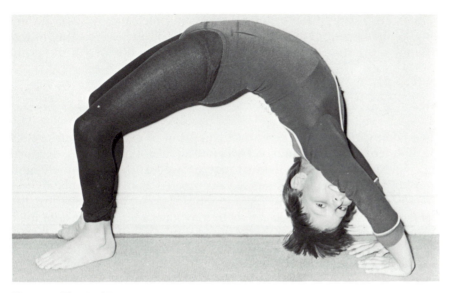

Fig. 8.17. The 'crab' position.

mainly employ hyperextension at the lumbar spine and the resultant position will have a high arch. Others, with a more rigid lumbar spine, will train for hyperextension at the shoulder and the hip and a greater range of hyperextension at these two joints will compensate for the relative lack of movement in the back. The resultant position has a flatter appearance and resembles a table top. In very stiff individuals it will be necessary to employ additional extension at the knees, wrists and ankle joints.

The extent to which mobility can be influenced by training was demonstrated in an investigation in which a pair of trained gymnasts both undertook the same position and the distance between their hands and feet was measured. Initially there was considerable variation between the two athletes and after a period of 10 min devoted to a series of exercises designed to further hyperextend the lumbar spine, the difference had become even more marked. One individual with a particularly supple spine was then able to walk her hands between her feet.

Swimming

Individuals prefer different strokes in accordance with their physical attribtues. The butterfly and crawl, for example, require a combination of flexibility and strength at the shoulder girdle, but the former stroke also demands considerable leg power. Newcomers are selected on the basis of their ability to perform these different swimming strokes and are trained accordingly.

Swimmers are aware of the beneficial effects of practising in warm water. The range of movement of joints is more rapidly and easily increased at the higher temperature than when participants exercise on the side of the pool.

Athletics

There is a wide variation in different activities, but in general athletes select their event in terms of body build. A small physique is suited to long-distance running, whereas the taller individual may do well at the long jump, high jump and hurdling. Several hurdlers have competed at an international level before having prosthetic hip joint replacement for premature osteoarthrosis. Acetabular dysplasia, inherited from birth, may have been the cause of their premature osteoarthrosis rather than the repetitive impulse loading that is characteristic of running but which has not been shown to accelerate damage in normal joints.

Modern techniques for high-jumping require great flexibility of the spine and hips and javelin throwers need similar attributes at the shoulder. Javelin throwers always use the same arm, which is not necessarily their dominant writing side. Some sportsmen have been known to throw the javelin with one hand but a cricket ball with the other.

Yoga

Some may be attracted to yoga for its philosophical content, but those who are more interested in physical improvement concentrate on the exercises, which may require a high degree of laxity. It is accepted in yoga that persons should only exercise within their own level of ability and that the final position achieved is immaterial. It follows that if all individuals subject themselves to approximately the same amount of training, different members of the same group will vary in the extent to which they can place their bodies in the standard yoga positions. In turn, this is likely to reflect their inherited laxity. In yoga the weight of the body is often supported by the floor, unlike ballet or gymnastics, where active muscle tone is necessary to hold the body in a relatively unsupported position.

Tennis

Tennis is an example of a sport that requires flexibility of the shoulder muscles and strength in the arms together with considerable neuromuscular co-ordination and good eyesight. Studies on students specialising in tennis at a physical education college suggest that muscle tone is more important than hyperextensibility of the shoulder.

Football

Hyperlaxity is not an advantage in football and studies performed on a professional football team have suggested that excessive mobility at the knee joint, particularly after operation, may be of considerable disadvantage. A modest degree of flexibility will help players to position the body when performing the sport to a high standard, but muscular co-ordination and strength in the lower limbs is the main requirement.

Cricket: Spin Bowling

The ability to impart spin on the cricket ball as it leaves the bowler's hand requires not only a high degree of lateral movement at the metacarpopha-langeal joints but also considerable neuromuscular co-ordination of the hand and fingers. It is analogous to the ability of a pianist to place chords of a wide spread with the inner fingers of the hand as the thumb and forefinger are extended at the octave or tenth. Studies with sportsmen at a physical education college suggest that this skill can in part be acquired. However, inherited factors may be important. In the epidemiological studies upon the range of movement at the fingers and metacarpophalangeal joints by the Leeds group, it was shown that Indians had a greater degree of laxity than Africans, who in turn were more mobile than Europeans. The sporting prowess of Indian spin-bowlers may be as much an inherited as an acquired trait, and it may not be for philosophical reasons alone that yoga evolved on the Indian sub-continent.

The Effect of Training on Joint Laxity in Sportsmen and Sportswomen

Familiarity with exercise regimes which will improve joint mobility is impor-tant to coaches and athletes in sports where a large range of movement is advantageous. In conjunction with Dr David Brodie, recently at Carnegie College of Physical Education, the Leeds group have evaluated a regular training programme designed to increase flexibility in a group of physical education students who were participating to a high standard in a large number of sports. The range of movement at all joints in the body was determined by goniometry, using the guidelines set out by the American Association of Orthopaedic Surgeons in a group of thirty physical education students with a mean age of 19 years. The class was then divided into two halves. One group daily used a series of flexibility exercises for half a term, about 5 weeks, while the other group continued with their normal sporting life. Measurements were taken at the end of this period and the two groups were then interchanged and remeasured after a further 5 weeks. The exercises performed, which had been recommended by physical education specialists, contrast, in the left hand, consisted of an initial warm-up period of 5 min, during which time subjects performed head rolling, side bending, arm swinging, trunk twisting and hip flexing. They then performed more arduous exercises in order to influence the flexibility of specific muscle groups.

Participants gradually increased the number of repetitions of each exercise performed over the period of the study and up to 15 min was spent on these exercises every day.

An analysis of results showed that a gradual though modest increase in flexibility had been achieved in almost all subjects. However, this increase was masked by the wide variation of natural movement that was present at the start of the study. As this particular group had been selected because of athletic prowess, their muscular strength and tone probably precluded a large change in mobility.

An attempt was also made to display the potential of exercises for increasing the range of movement. Four females with marked hypermobility continued with the same exercises for a further period of 7 weeks at a more arduous and advanced level. Measurements designed to detect change both in trunk and hip mobility were carried out at weekly intervals. Only one displayed a serial increase in joint laxity, another showed slight reduction, while two showed an intermediate picture with improvement occurring in only certain movements. It is clear that no single set of exercises would be appropriate to all individuals. There is a wide variation between subjects in the increase in range of joint movement that can be attained by regular training.

Although this study was limited to a group of selected athletes, there are important clinical implications in the possible effects of physiotherapy on patients with rheumatic diseases. Inherited and acquired joint laxity may both be altered by physiotherapy. Account must also be taken of the damage that has occurred to both joints and muscles before an improvement can be ascribed to any one type of therapy.

References

Ballet Dancers

Beighton P (1970) The Ehlers–Danlos syndrome, William Heinemann Medical Books, London

Burry HC, Grahame R (1973) The role of physical therapy in the treatment of soft tissue injury. Trans Med Soc Lond 89: 241–247

El Sayed TF, Hilson AJW, Maisey MN, Saunders AJS, Grahame R (1979) Stress lesions of the lower leg and foot. Clin Radiol 30: 649–654

Grahame R, Jenkins JM (1972) Joint hypermobility—asset or liability? A study of joint mobility in ballet dancers. Ann Rheum Dis 31: 109–111

Grahame R, Saunders AS, Maisey MN (1979) The use of scintigraphy in the diagnosis and management of traumatic foot lesions in ballet dancers. Rheum Rehab 18: 235–238

Miller EH, Schneider HJ, Bronson JL, McLain D (1975) A new consideration in athletic injuries. The classical ballet dancer. Clin Orthop 111: 181–195

Schneider HJ, King AY, Bronson JL, Miller EH (1974) Stress injuries and developmental change of lower extremities of ballet dancers. Radiology 113: 627–632

Washington EL (1978) Musculo-skeletal injuries in theatrical dancers. Site, frequency and severity. Am J Sports Med 6 (2): 75–97

Musicians

Bird HA, Wright V (1981) Traumatic synovitis in a classical guitarist: the study of joint laxity. Ann Rheum Dis 40: 161–163

Jobbins B, Bird HA, Wright V (1979) A joint hyperextensometer for the quantification of joint laxity. Eng Med 8: 103–104

Inherited Hypermobility Syndromes

Key to Pedigree

Symbols used in Pedigrees (Figs. 9.10; 9.11; 10.5; 10.6)

☐   Normal male   ⊙   Carrier female

◯   Normal female   \   Deceased

■   Affected male   ↖   Proband

●   Affected female

9. Ehlers–Danlos Syndrome

Introduction

The Ehlers–Danlos syndrome (EDS) is an inherited disorder of connective tissue which is characterised by the clinical triad of articular hypermobility, dermal extensibility and cutaneous scarring. The manifestations are very variable although usually fairly consistent within any kindred, and it has become increasingly evident that EDS is very heterogeneous.

The joint laxity in EDS leads to a wide variety of rheumatological complications; these are discussed in detail in this chapter and other relevant facets are reviewed in terms of current concepts. Detailed accounts of the condition can be found in a monograph 'The Ehlers–Danlos syndrome' by Beighton (1970) and in the classical work 'Heritable disorders of connective tissue' (McKusick 1972).

EDS is of topical interest because of the protean nature of its clinical complications, the unfolding heterogeneity and the recognition of the biochemical defect in some forms of the disorder. A selective bibliography of recent publications which are of fundamental importance or rheumatological interest is given at the end of this chapter.

Historical Background

The first recognisable description of EDS concerned a young Spaniard, George Albes, who was exhibited before the Academy of Leyden in 1657, by the Dutch surgeon Job Janszoon van Meek'ren. Albes was able to stretch the skin of his chest so that it covered his eyes. In the days of the fairground peep show a number of persons with the syndrome made their living by demonstrating their excessive cutaneous extensibility. Perhaps the most famous was Etta Lake, the 'Elastic Lady', who is depicted in Fig. 9.1.

The initial scientific appraisal of the condition is credited to Chernogubov, who demonstrated an affected 17-year-old Russian boy at the Moscow Venereology and Dermatology Society in 1892. In a translation of the original paper, Denko (1978) pointed out that in the Soviet Union the condition is still

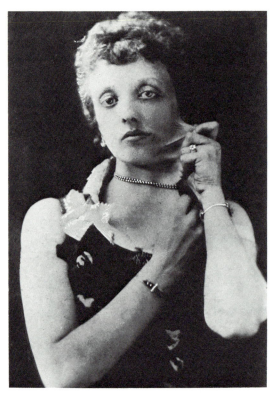

Fig. 9.1. Etta Lake, the 'Elastic Lady'. Miss Lake was a professional exhibitionist who toured Europe and North America about 50 years ago. This photograph was found in a fairground peepshow. Mr Tim Bowman, the owner of the show and the grandson of Etta's former manager gave his kind permission for the illustration to be published.

known as 'Chernogubov's syndrome'. Thereafter the disorder gained its eponymous title and achieved medical recognition following the early case reports by Ehlers (1901) and Danlos (1908).

The terminology became complex in the early part of the 20th century and many titles which were descriptive of the various features of the syndrome were employed. Among these were dermatorrhexis, dermatolysis, gummi-haut, cutis pendula, cutis hyperelastica and chalasodermia. However, lax skin and loose joints also exist as isolated entities, and there was therefore a great deal of confusion. Parkes Weber tried to delineate these conditions, and pointed out that skin hyperextensibility and fragility, together with joint laxity and molluscoid pseudo-tumours, had been described in the original patients, and that the eponym 'Ehlers–Danlos' was appropriate to the disorder.

The condition was diagnosed with increasing frequency, and the first large review was published by Ronchese (1936) of Rhode Island, who located 24 patients in the literature and added three of his own. When McKusick compiled his monograph in 1956, there were less than 100 case reports, but by the beginning of 1982 more than 500 affected persons had been reported in over 300 articles. Heterogeneity has been increasingly recognised and more than ten different forms of the disorder have now been delineated. The majority of these are rare but the establishment of their syndromic identity is warranted, as their biochemical defects have been discovered in most instances. A problem of classification is now arising due to this proliferation of subtypes of EDS, and the currently accepted syndromic boundaries require reappraisal.

General Features

There is considerable variation in the extent to which individuals may be affected by EDS, and the clinical manifestations and complications are by no means consistent. However, the components of the diagnostic triad of extensible skin, loose joints and fragile tissues are always present in some degree (Figs. 9.2, 9.3 and 9.4).

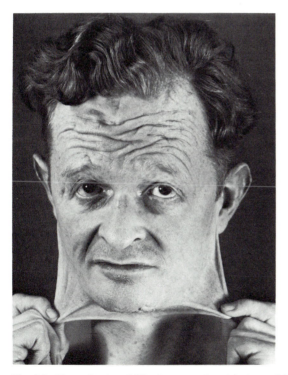

Fig. 9.2. Dermal extensibility is a prominent feature of EDS. On release the skin springs back to take up its former position.

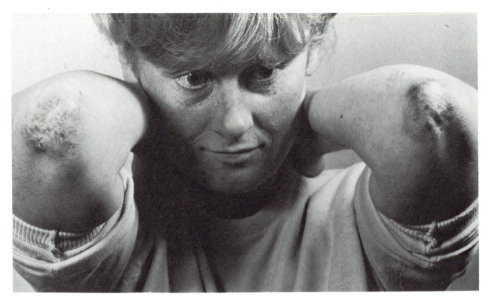

Fig. 9.3. Thin pigmented scars over the bony prominences result from trivial trauma.

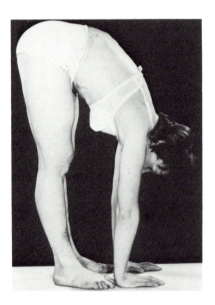

Fig. 9.4. Articular hypermobility is variable in degree, but often very marked.

The skin splits on minor trauma, forming gaping lacerations. These heal slowly and wide papyraceous scars develop which are often darkly pigmented and are typically found over the knees and elbows. Raisin-like swellings known as molluscoid pseudo-tumours are often present in scarred areas and hard calcified subcutaneous spheroids may be palpated in the forearms and shins.

Scars on the forehead and chin usually have a linear configuration (Fig. 9.5). Epicanthic folds and lop ears are other features which contribute to the characteristic facies.

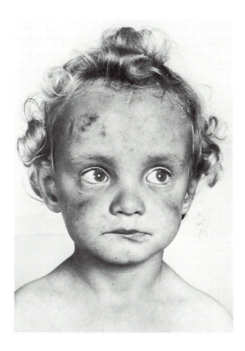

Fig. 9.5. EDS I (gravis type). An infant with the characteristic linear scars on the forehead.

In addition to the dermatological problems, complications are encountered in virtually every system of the body. These have a common basis in connective tissue extensibility and fragility. In a minority of patients, notably those with EDS type IV, sudden death occurs from rupture of large arteries (McFarland and Fuller 1964; Wright et al. 1979), dissection of the aorta (Beighton 1968) or gastrointestinal perforation and bleeding (Beighton et al. 1969).

A bleeding tendency is a very variable feature of EDS. At one end of the spectrum, abnormal bleeding may lead to a spurious diagnosis of haemophilia, while at the other, the clotting mechanism is apparently normal. The nature of this problem has not been elucidated, but platelet abnormalities have been implicated (Kashiwagi et al. 1965; Estes 1966; Onel et al. 1973).

Nosology

Heterogeneity was initially suspected on clinical and genetic grounds (Barabas 1967; Beighton 1968, 1970; Beighton et al. 1969). Further delineation was achieved by the recognition of the basic biochemical abnormality in a number of patients. The nomenclature and mode of inheritance of the various forms of EDS are given in Table 9.1. The major clinical features are also listed and those of EDS types I–V are depicted in Figs. 9.6–9.10. Pedigrees of families with the common autosomal dominant EDS type II (mitis) and the rare X-linked EDS type V are shown in Figs. 9.11 and 9.12. Heterogeneity has been postulated in type IV EDS (Pope et al. 1980).

The concept of heterogeneity in type IV EDS is supported by differing ultrastructural changes in the dermis which have been identified by Byers et al. (1979) and Sulica et al. (1979).

Table 9.1. The different forms of EDS

Type	Skin hyperextensibility	Joint hypermobility	Skin splitting
I Gravis	Gross	Gross	Gross
II Mitis	Moderate	Moderate	Moderate
III Benign hypermobile	Variable, usually gross	Gross	Minimal
IV Ecchymotic	Minimal	Minimal	Moderate
V X-linked	Moderate	Moderate	Minimal
VI Ocular	Moderate	Moderate	Moderate
VII Arthrocholasis multiplex congenita	Moderate	Gross	Minimal

Type	Bruising	Inheritance	Major concomitants
I Gravis	Moderate	AD	Musculo-skeletal deformity, varicose veins, prematurity?
II Mitis	Moderate	AD	
III Benign hypermobile	Minimal	AD	
IV Ecchymotic	Gross	AD/AR	Death from arterial rupture
V X-linked	Minimal	XL	
VI Ocular	Moderate	AR	Ocular fragility with scleral rupture and retinal detachment
VII Arthrocholasis multiplex congenita	Moderate	AR	Multiple dislocations, short stature, depressed nasal bridge

AD = autosomal dominant
AR = autosomal recessive
XL = X-linked

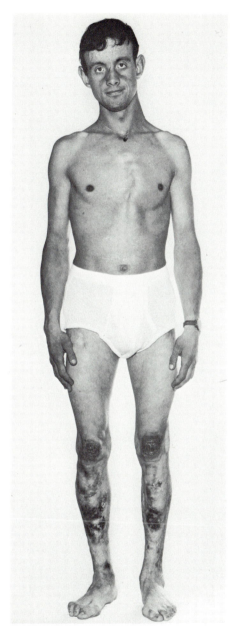

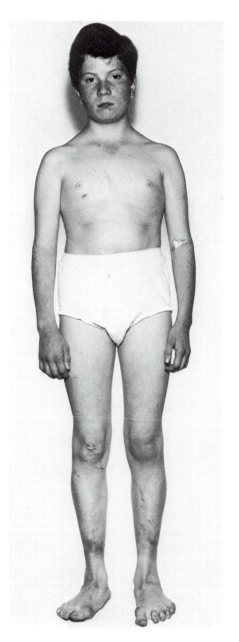

Fig. 9.6. The patient depicted in Fig. 9.5 20 years later. The manifestations are severe and the cutaneous fragility has led to widespread scarring. Pes planus, hallux valgus and claw toes are the consequences of gross articular hypermobility.

Fig. 9.7. EDS II (mitis type). The joint laxity, dermal extensibility and connective tissue fragility are mild and complications are infrequent in this form of EDS.

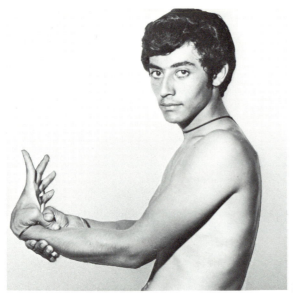

Fig. 9.8.

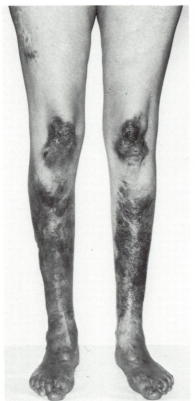

Fig. 9.9.

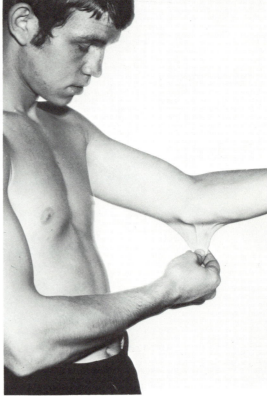

Fig. 9.10.

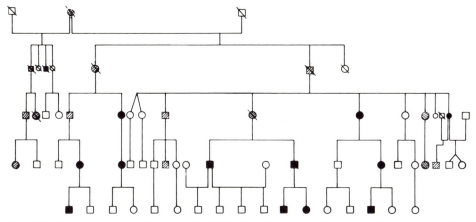

Fig. 9.11. A pedigree of a family with EDS II (mitis type). The generation to generation transmission and the ratio of affected and unaffected individuals is in accordance with autosomal dominant inheritance.

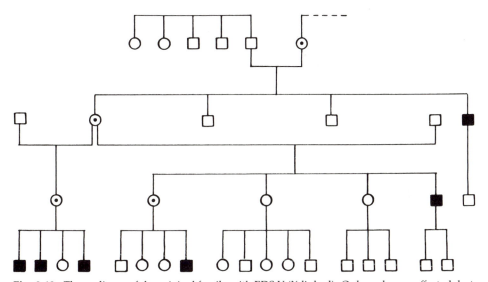

Fig. 9.12. The pedigree of the original family with EDS V (X-linked). Only males are affected, but clinically normal 'carrier' females can transmit the gene to their sons.

◀ *Opposite*

Fig. 9.8. EDS III (benign hypermobile type). Articular hypermobility is pronounced and a moderate degree of dermal extensibility is present, but there is little or no tendency to skin splitting or scarring.

Fig. 9.9. EDS IV (arterial or ecchymotic type). The bruising tendency is severe and the cutaneous scars are darkly pigmented. Joint mobility and dermal extensibility are not pronounced. This form of EDS is potentially lethal, due to spontaneous rupture of the large blood vessels or perforation of the intestinal wall.

Fig. 9.10. EDS V (X-linked type). In EDS V the articular laxity and cutaneous fragility and extensibility are all of moderate degree. As this form of the condition is X-linked, only males are affected. Females who carry the faulty gene do not have any clinical stigmata.

The biochemical defects in the comparatively common EDS types I, II and III are unknown, but the abnormalities which have been detected in the other rare types are listed in Table 9.2.

Table 9.2. Biochemical defects in EDS

Type	Synonym	Inheritance	Biochemical abnormality	Reference
EDS IV	Ecchymotic or arterial	AR	Unknown	
	Acrogeria	AR/AD	Type III collagen deficiency (total or variable)	Pope et al. (1975, 1977)
EDS V	X-linked	XL	Lysyl oxidase deficiency	Di Ferrante et al. (1975)
			Normal lysyl oxidase levels	Siegel et al. (1979)
EDS VI	Ocular	AR	Hydroxylysine-deficient collagen (lysyl hydroxylase deficiency)	Pinnell et al. (1972)
EDS VII	Arthrocholasis multiplex congenita	AR	Procollagen peptidase deficiency	Lichtenstein et al. (1974)
		AR	Extension peptide mutation	B Steinemann (cited by Pope et al. 1980)

An autosomal dominant 'periodontic' type of EDS was described by Stewart et al. (1977) and listed in 'Mendelian inheritance in man' (McKusick 1978) as 'EDS VIII'. Nelson and King (1981) subsequently reported a family with three affected members whom they considered to have the same disorder. The situation is confused, as the designation 'EDS VIII' was also used by Behrens-Baumann et al. (1977) for a form of EDS VI in which lysyl hydroxylation was normal. McKusick (1978) suggested that it might be appropriate to subdivide this latter category into 'EDS VI A and EDS VI B', but the matter remains unsettled.

There seems to be no end to heterogeneity in the condition; Beasley and Cohen (1979) reported a mentally retarded Chinese brother and sister with a variance of EDS in which marked hypermobility had led to bilateral hip dislocation. Their unaffected parents were consanguineous, and autosomal recessive inheritance was proposed.

Hernandez et al. (1979) described two young Mexican males with a form of EDS in which mental retardation, short stature, wrinkled facies, scanty eyebrows, periodontitis and multiple naevi were associated with the usual stigmata of the syndrome. A third case was added in a further report (Hernandez et al. 1981). The authors pointed out that the paternal age was increased in each instance, and speculated that their patients might be new mutants for an autosomal dominant gene.

A putative 'EDS IX' has recently been delineated by Arneson et al. (1980) in a sister and her three brothers who had the classical stigmata of EDS with defective activity of the adhesive glycoprotein 'fibronectin'. Due to this deficiency, cell to cell adhesion and aggregation of platelets with collagen was impaired. The parents and two other siblings were normal and inheritance was probably autosomal recessive.

Current interest is centred on the delineation of new forms of EDS on the basis of their biochemical abnormalities. However, it cannot be emphasised too strongly that more than 80% of all EDS patients have type I and II forms and that a further 10% have type III. Paradoxically, their fundamental defect is unknown, although it is these entities which are likely to be encountered in clinical practice.

Articular Manifestations

Hypermobility of the joints is a cardinal manifestation of EDS and articular problems are frequently encountered. The complications which were present in a series of 100 patients of all ages (Beighton and Horan 1969a) are listed in Table 9.3.

These patients were a heterogeneous group, but the majority had the severe gravis type I or mild mitis type II EDS, and the figures quoted above must be regarded in that light.

Dislocations

The degree of articular hypermobility and the incidence of dislocations are closely related, although in some persons a surprising range of joint movement can occur without causing clinical problems (Fig. 9.13). The joints most frequently affected are those of the digits, elbows, shoulders and patella, while dislocation of the sterno-clavicular joints has also been recorded. Congenital dislocation of the hips occurs in a minority of patients. A single instance of chronic temporomandibular joint subluxation has been reported (Goodman and Allison 1969).

Dislocations are often recurrent but reduction is usually easy and often spontaneous, particularly in the digital and shoulder joints. The degree of hypermobility and the incidence of dislocations usually lessens with ageing. However, there may be a temporary increase in the liability to dislocation during pregnancy.

Table 9.3. Complications in EDS

Complication	Number of patients
Dislocations—26 patients	
Digits and thumbs	7
Elbows	3
Shoulder joint	13
Temporomandibular joint	2
Patella	8
Congenital dislocation hip	1
Hip	1
Effusions—20 patients	
Knee	15
Ankle	4
Elbows	3
Digits	2
Joint instability—20 patients	
Ankle	11
Knee	6
Other	3
Osteoarthritis—20 patients	
Severe incapacity from widespread O.A.	2
Knees (unilateral)	10
Hands	5
Ankles	2
Shoulder (bilateral)	1
Spinal Abnormality—23 patients	
Scoliosis	18
Thoraco-lumbar kyphosis	6
Straight thoracic spine	2
Thoracic cage abnormality	
Depressed sternum	8
Prominence of costochondral junctions	8
Minor degrees of thoracic asymmetry	14
Foot deformity	
Talipes equinovarus	7
Pes planus	52
Muscle cramps	43
Raynaud's phenomenon	7
Acrocyanosis	20

Joint Instability

The more hypermobile patients are frequently troubled by instability of the joints, particularly the ankles and the knees (Figs. 9.14 and 9.15). For this reason, such activities as running or the wearing of high heels may be impossible. Instability of the finger joints may also be a problem and simple actions like typing or unscrewing bottle tops may be very difficult.

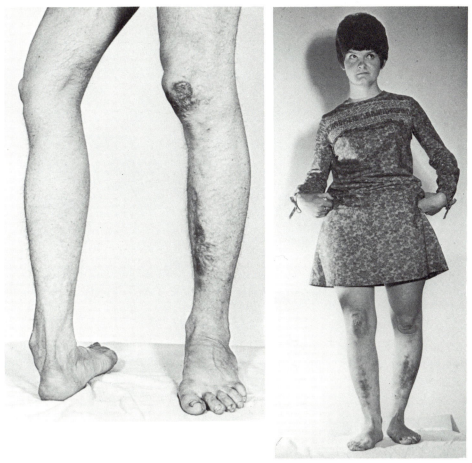

Fig. 9.13. (*left*) In some persons with the EDS, articular laxity may be extreme and it is not surprising that a large variety of musculo-skeletal complications may occur.

Fig. 9.14. (*right*) An affected girl with instability of the knee and ankle. Her shins bear the characteristic scars.

It must be stressed that not all patients are troubled by joint instability. Amongst persons known to have EDS are a racing cyclist, a weight-lifter and an amateur boxing champion.

Joint Effusions

Persistent or recurrent effusions are commonly encountered. The usual site is the knee joint, but the ankles, elbows and digits may also be affected. Effusions seem to be related to activity and commonly appear at the end of the day. Although the joints are not excessively mobile in the X-linked form of EDS, effusions are a particular feature of this variety of the condition.

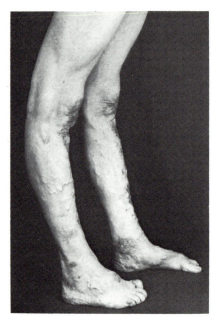

Fig. 9.15. Articular laxity may lead to marked genu recurvatum.

Haemarthroses may occur in a minority of patients in whom the bleeding tendency is severe. A misdiagnosis of haemophilia has been made on occasion.

Hypotonicity

Many individuals have muscular hypotonicity, which is probably directly associated with their lax joints. In infancy, the recognition of EDS may be very difficult, particularly as all babies are somewhat hypermobile. EDS should certainly be considered in the differential diagnosis of any 'floppy infant', as a misdiagnosis of Oppenheim's disease and Werdnig–Hoffman disease has been made in several affected newborn babies.

Spinal Abnormalities

Spinal abnormalities of greater or lesser degree may be present in a significant proportion of patients. Thoraco-lumbar scoliosis is the commonest abnormality of this type, and vertebral wedging may occur at the apex of the kyphotic element of the curve when a severe scoliosis is present. In a few patients, the thoracic spine has been remarkably straight.

The fact that spinal changes are uncommon in affected children suggests that the scoliosis is caused by the strains imposed by the upright stance on vertebral joints which have lax ligaments.

Thoracic Asymmetry

Asymmetry of the thorax and sternal depression may occur, particularly in conjunction with spinal deformities. When severe, the thoracic deformity may cause displacement of the heart, which in turn can lead to a cardiac murmur and an abnormal electrocardiogram.

Foot Deformities

Talipes equinovarus is present at birth in about 7% of persons with EDS (Fig. 9.16). As intrauterine malposition may be a causative factor in the pathogenesis of club foot, it is reasonable to postulate that individuals with abnormally mobile joints would be at an unusually high risk for this complication. This hypothesis would explain the high incidence of talipes in patients with EDS.

Pes planus is a consistent abnormality, occurring in many affected patients. In younger individuals the longitudinal arch frequently appears to be normal when no weight is being borne, but by the age of 30 the majority of patients with flat feet show both static and dynamic pes planus deformity (Fig. 9.17). These changes are maximal in the more hypermobile patients. The most severe flat feet usually give no pain, and difficulty in fitting shoes is the main problem.

Hallux valgus, claw toes and plantar keratomata are other common problems in the feet. The extensible skin may contribute to an appearance of 'moccasin feet' where the patient seems to be wearing an oversize pair of ankle socks.

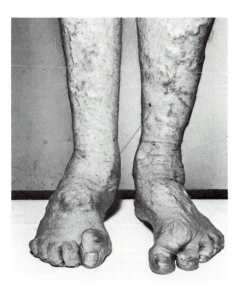

Fig. 9.16. The feet of the patient depicted in Fig. 9.2. Talipes equinovarus which was present at birth had been corrected surgically but his feet were still deformed.

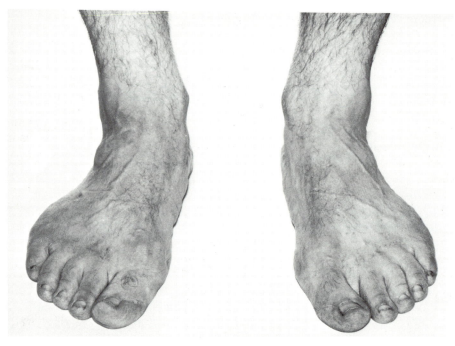

Fig. 9.17. The majority of persons with EDS have pes planus on weight bearing.

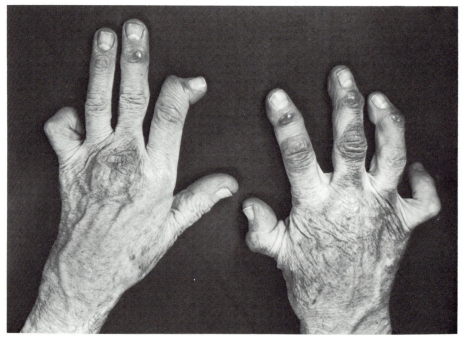

Fig. 9.18. In severely affected individuals digital deformities may result from repeated subluxa-tions and dislocations.

Osteoarthritis

The development of osteoarthritis appears to be directly related to the magnitude of hypermobility and the frequency and degree of trauma to which a particular joint is exposed (Figs. 9.18 and 9.19). Osteoarthritis has been observed in the hands, knees, ankles and shoulders, and the majority of patients are affected by the age of 40. However, there are no reports of osteoarthritis of the hip joint. Backache is surprisingly uncommon in view of the high incidence of spinal deformities (Figs. 9.20 and 9.21).

Osborn et al. (1981) studied nine children with EDS type II or III who presented with painful joints and suggested that the condition warranted consideration in the differential diagnosis of any child with polyarthralgia.

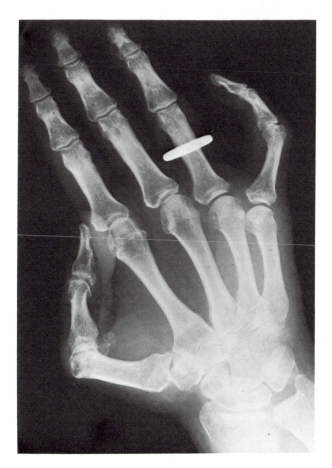

Fig. 9.19. A hand radiograph of an elderly lady with EDS showing generalised osteoarthritis.

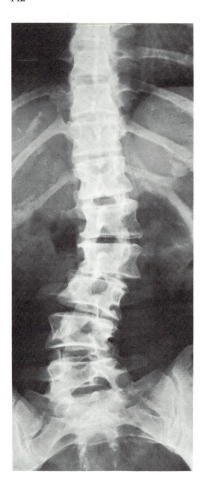

Fig. 9.20. Lateral radiograph of the lumbar spine of a middle-aged patient with malalignment and osteoarthritis.

Bursae

Bursae may develop in association with the tendo-Achilles, hallux valgus, and in the olecranon and pre-patella regions. It is sometimes difficult to distinguish these bursae from haematomata or from molluscoid pseudo-tumours, which also occur at these sites. The results of excision of these bursae are usually good.

Muscle Cramps

A considerable proportion of patients experience cramps in their calf muscles. These usually occur at night and are most severe during childhood, often resolving completely in adult life. The pathogenesis is unknown, but it is

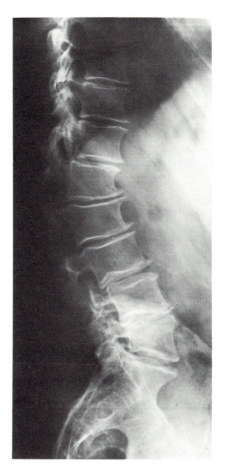

Fig. 9.21. Antero-posterior radiograph of the spine of young woman with EDS, showing marked scoliosis in the lumbar region.

tempting to speculate that they are caused by the overstretching of the muscles which is permitted by the abnormal range of movements of the lax joints. Bilkey et al. (1981) carried out extensive muscle function studies in a young woman with EDS and demonstrated a functional proprioceptive deficit in the absence of any inherent muscle abnormality.

Peripheral Circulatory Phenomena

Acrocyanosis occurs in many patients, while a substantial minority experience Raynaud's phenomenon. Chilblains are common, particularly during childhood. Acro-osteolysis has been described in a French girl (Mabille et al. 1971) and there is an instance of a middle-aged English woman with the same problem.

Bony Features

A variety of bony features have been encountered in isolated cases, including radio-ulnar synostosis, lack of development of the proximal phalanx of the little finger, syndactyly, spina bifida occulta, and abnormalities of cranial ossification. However, it is unlikely that these changes are directly related to EDS, as a majority of patients do not have any significant primary bony abnormality. Rao (1979) reported monostotic fibrous dysplasia in a child with EDS; again it is difficult to put forward any unitary hypothesis to explain this concurrence. The incidence of fractures is no higher than in normal individuals, and their healing is uneventful. There is no increased liability to musculo-skeletal neoplasia.

Handshake

Affected individuals have a characteristic handshake. The musculoskeletal structure of the hand seems to collapse on pressure and the hand feels like a bag of bones.

Gait

Patients can often be recognised by their gait. The feet are placed firmly and flatly upon the ground. The hips are hyperextended during weight-bearing to counteract the genu recurvatum, thus enabling the pelvis to remain balanced with respect to the feet. This gait is accentuated by the concomitant pes planus, and resembles that of tabes dorsalis.

Surgical Management of Articular Problems

The majority of complications which involve the joints respond to conventions of EDS. They are probably due to distensibility and fragility of the made difficult by a series of potential hazards. These have been reviewed by Beighton and Horan (1969b) and Bennett (1977) amongst others.

Surgical procedures may be complicated by the fragility of the tissues. Sutures often cut out and closure of operation sites may be difficult. Surgeons have aptly described attempts at skin suture as being 'like trying to sew porridge (Hulme and Wilmshurst 1976). Similarly, angiographic procedures have caused major lacerations of the femoral artery. However, the majority of patients do not have operative problems of this magnitude.

A bleeding tendency may be present in some individuals. Although the majority of patients have trouble-free operations, massive haemorrhage has occurred in a few instances. The bleeding diathesis has been variously ascribed to changes in the coagulation mechanism, vessel walls or perivascular connective tissues. However, no consistent abnormality has been demonstrated.

Post-operative haematoma formation may delay wound healing. The diminution of tissue elasticity, which would usually prevent the expansion of such haematomata, is probably significant.

Due to the tissue fragility a small skin incision may extend spontaneously to become a gaping wound. The deeper tissues are also fragile and as sutures often tear out, closure may be difficult. Fine suture material, the avoidance of tension and a meticulous technique increases the chances of satisfactory operative results.

Healing is often slow and wounds may re-open when sutures are removed. Surgical scars are usually thin and they frequently widen and distract with the passage of time, even when initial healing has been satisfactory.

A Patient's Viewpoint of His Articular Problems

A young man with EDS wrote the following excellent description of certain aspects of his condition.

My skin is rather loose and my knee joints will extend about 2″ further back than a normal person's knees. If I stand with my knees straight I have to use my leg muscles to hold them there. If I let my knees extend backwards to their locked position it doesn't take long until they ache from the awkward position which they are in. The weight of my body rests on my knees at a slight angle from the vertical, which results in a strain being put upon them. Not only is my skin loose but the supporting tissue under the skin is soft. Although I am a construction electrician and work with my hands, I do not form callouses on them. Sometimes when I lift something heavy I feel the tissue give way between the bones of my fingers and the object that I am lifting.

Non-articular Complications

Apart from the articular complications, a wide variety of problems in other systems may arise from the underlying connective tissue abnormality. These are briefly reviewed below.

Cardiological

Structural cardiac defects were initially thought not to be a fundamental feature of EDS. However, as in other inherited disorders of connective tissue, a 'floppy mitral valve' is not uncommon and with the introduction of sophisticated investigation techniques a variety of cardiac abnormalities have been recognised (Cabeen et al. 1977; Leier et al. 1980).

The potentially lethal complications of dissection of the aorta and spontaneous rupture of large arteries are virtually confined to the very rare type IV (arterial form) of EDS.

Gastrointestinal

Structural anomalies of the gastrointestinal tract result from the undue tissue laxity. These abnormalities include hiatus hernia, gastric, duodenal and colonic diverticulae, and rectal prolapse. Inguinal, femoral and umbilical herniae are also common.

Gastrointestinal haemorrhage, with or without perforation, is a feature of the rare EDS type IV. These events may be spontaneous, or follow minor trauma, and several deaths have been reported.

Neurological

Intracranial vascular abnormalities are uncommon but dangerous complications of EDS. They are probably due to distensibility and fragility of the walls of the blood vessels, and the problems which arise are compounded by the bleeding tendency. Aneurysms of the internal carotid arteries, carotid-cavernous sinus fistulae and subarachnoid haemorrhage have all been reported. Angiographic investigation of intracranial lesions of this type are hazardous.

Haematomata may compress peripheral nerves. Spinal malalignment can result in cord compression, but this complication is rare.

Ophthalmological

Involvement of the scleral connective tissue permits distortion of the eyeball and myopia is present in a proportion of patients. These individuals may develop a divergent strabismus, but uncomplicated convergent squint is more common. This latter complication has been attributed to laxity of the tendons of the extrinsic muscles of the eye. Scleral perforation and potential visual loss are features of the rare type VI EDS.

Epicanthic folds and redundant skin on the upper eyelid may produce undesirable cosmetic effects. In this context, Metenier's sign (ease of eversion of the upper eyelid) is one of the minor diagnostic features of EDS.

Obstetric

The tissue fragility and bleeding tendency pose special hazards during pregnancy, and expert antenatal care and delivery are desirable. In one horrific episode, forceps delivery in an affected woman resulted in extraction of the infant, together with the uterus, bladder and ureters.

Antepartum and postpartum haemorrhage are not infrequent, and it may be difficult to achieve haemostasis. Precipitate labour, severe perianal lacerations and uterine prolapse are relatively common. If the foetus has inherited the condition, the amniotic and chorionic membranes will be fragile. These may rupture at an early stage, causing premature labour.

One aspect of EDS which is regarded as advantageous by affected females is the fact that striae gravidarum do not develop during pregnancy!

Comment

As laboratory methods for the investigation of collagen biochemistry become increasingly sophisticated, it is probable that further forms of EDS will be delineated. Until now these investigations have pertained to the rare types of the EDS, but the revolutionary developments in recombinant DNA technology will be applicable to the common varieties and the fundamental molecular defect may ultimately be elucidated. This will have important implications for diagnostic categorisation and perhaps for antenatal diagnosis.

In spite of the application of sophisticated technology, the individual patient is still concerned with clinical problems. Perhaps the last word should rest with the young lady with EDS, who complained 'when I was a baby they called me a floppy infant, and now the doctors tell me that I am a loose woman'!

References

Arneson MA, Hammerschmidt DE, Furcht LT, King RA (1980) A new form of Ehlers–Danlos syndrome: fibronectin corrects defective platelet function. JAMA 224: 144–147

Barabas AP (1967) Heterogeneity of the Ehlers–Danlos syndrome: Description of three clinical types and a hypothesis to explain the basic defect(s). Br Med J 2: 612–616

Beasley RP, Cohen MM (1979) A new presumably autosomal recessive form of the Ehlers–Danlos syndrome. Clin Genet 16: 19–24

Behrens-Baumann W, Gebauer HJ, Langenbeck U (1977) syndrome of blue sclerae and keratoglobus (ocular type of Ehlers–Danlos syndrome). Arch Klin Opthalmol 204(4): 235–246

Beighton P (1968) X-Linked recessive inheritance in the Ehlers–Danlos syndrome. Br Med J 3: 409–414

Beighton P (1968) Lethal complications of the Ehlers–Danlos syndrome. Br Med J 3: 656–660

Beighton P, Horan F (1969a) Orthopaedic aspects of the Ehlers–Danlos syndrome. J Bone Joint Surg [Br] 513: 414–449

Beighton P, Horan F (1969b) Surgical aspects of the Ehlers–Danlos syndrome. Br J Surg 56: 255–259

Beighton P, Murdoch JL, Votteler T (1969) Gastrointestinal complications of the Ehlers–Danlos syndrome. Gut 10: 1004–1008

Beighton P, Price A, Lord A, Dickson E (1969) Variants of the Ehlers–Danlos syndrome. Clinical, biochemical, haematological and chromosomal features of 100 patients. Ann Rheum Dis 28: 228–235

Beighton P (1970) The Ehlers–Danlos syndrome. William Heinemann Medical Books, London

Beighton P (1970) Serious ophthalmological complications in the Ehlers–Danlos syndrome. Br J Ophthalmol 54: 263–269

Bennett JB (1977) Flexor tendon laceration in Ehlers–Danlos syndrome. A case report. J Bone Joint Surg 59(2): 259–260

Bilkey WJ, Baxter TL, Kottke FJ, Mundale MO (1981) Muscle formation in Ehlers–Danlos syndrome. Arch Phys Med Rehabil 62(9): 444–448

Byers PH, Holbrook KA, McGillivray B, MacLeod PM, Lowry RB (1979) Clinical and ultrastructural heterogeneity of type IV Ehlers–Danlos syndrome. Hum Genet 47(2): 141–150

Cabeen WR, Reza MJ, Kovick RB Stern MS (1977) Mitral valve prolapse and conduction defects in Ehlers–Danlos syndrome. Arch Intern Med 137(9): 1227–1231

Danlos M (1908) Un cas de cutis Laxa avec tumeurs par contusion chronique des coudes et des genoux (Xanthome juvenile pseudodiabetique de M.M. Hallopeau et Mace de Lepinay). Bull Soc Franc Derm Syph 19: 70–72

Denko CW (1978) Chernogubov's syndrome: A translation of the first modern case report of the Ehlers–Danlos syndrome. J Rheum 5(3): 347–352

Di Ferrante N, Leachman RD, Angelini P, Donnelly PV, Francis G, Almazan A, Segni G (1975) Lysyl oxidase deficiency in Ehlers–Danlos syndrome type V. Connect Tissue Res 3: 49–53

Ehlers E (1901) Cutis Laxa, Niegung zu Haemorrhagien in der Haut, Lockerung Mehrer Artikulationen. Derm Z 8: 173–175

Estes JW (1968) Platelet size and function in the heritable disorders of connective tissue. Ann Intern Med 68: 1237–1249

Goodman RM, Allison ML, (1969) Chronic temporomandibular joint subluxation in Ehlers–Danlos syndrome: report of case. J Oral Surg 27: 659–661

Hernandez A, Aguirre–Negrete MG, Ramirez–Soltero S, Gonzalez–Mendoza A, Martinez y Martinez R, Velazquez–Cabrera A, Cantu JM (1979) A distinct variant of the Ehlers–Danlos syndrome. Clin Genet 16: 335–339

Hernandez A, Aguirre–Negrete MG, Liparoli JC, Canto JM (1981) Third case of a distinct variant of the Ehlers–Danlos syndrome (EDS). Clin Genet 20: 222–224

Hulme JR, Wilmshurst CC (1976) Acute appendicitis in the Ehlers–Danlos syndrome. Am J Surg 132: 103–104

Kashiwagi H, Riddle JM, Abraham JP, Frame B (1965) Functional and ultrastructural abnormalities of platelets in Ehlers–Danlos syndrome. Ann Intern Med 63: 249–254

Leier CV, Call TD, Fulkerson PK, Wooley CF (1980) The spectrum of cardiac defects in the Ehlers–Danlos syndrome, types I and III. Ann Intern Med 92(2 Pt 1): 171–178

Lichtenstein JR, Martin GR, Kohn LD, Byers PH, McKusick VA (1974) Defect in conversion of procollagen in a form of Ehlers–Danlos syndrome. Science 182: 298–300

Mabille JP, Castera D, Chapuis JL, Lambert D, Chapelion (1972) Un cas de syndrome d'Ehlers–Danlos avec acro-osteolyse. Ann Radiol 15(9-10): 781–786

McFarland W, Fuller DE (1964) Mortality in Ehlers–Danlos syndrome due to spontaneous rupture of large arteries. N Engl Med 271: 1309–1312

McKusick VA (1972) Heritable disorders of connective tissue, 4th edn. CV Mosby Co, St Louis Baltimore

McKusick VA (1978) Mendelian inheritance in man, 5th edn. Johns Hopkins University Press,

Nelson DL, King RA (1981) Ehlers–Danlos syndrome type VIII. J Am Acad Dermatol 5(3): 297–303

Onel D, Ulutin SB, Ulutin ON (1973) Platelet defect in a case of Ehlers–Danlos syndrome. Acta Haematol 50(4): 238–244

Osborn TG, Lichenstein JR, Moore TL, Weiss T, Zuckner J (1981) Ehlers–Danlos syndrome presenting as rheumatic manifestations in the child. J Rheumatol 8(1): 79–85

Pinnell SR, Krane SM, Kenzora JE, Glimcher A (1972) A heritable disorder of connective tissue: hydroxylysine deficient collagen disease. N Engl J Med 286: 1013–1020

Pope FM, Martin GR, Lichenstein JR Penttinen R, Gerson B, Rowe DW (1975) Patients with Ehlers–Danlos syndrome type IV lack type III collagen. Proc Natl Acad Sci USA 72: 1314–1316

Pope FM, Martin GR, McKusick VA (1977) Inheritance of Ehlers–Danlos type IV syndrome. J Med Genet 14: 200–204

Pope FM, Jones PM, Wells RS, Lawrence D (1980) EDS IV (acrogeria): new autosomal dominant and recessive types. J R Soc Med 73: 180–186

Rao AA (1979) Ehlers–Danlos syndrome with monostotic fibrous dysplasia. J Postgrad Med 25(3): 186–188

Ronchese F (1936) Dermatorrhexis with Dermatochalasis and Arthrochalasis (the so-called Ehlers–Danlos Syndrome). Am J Dis Child 51: 1403–1406

Siegel RC, Black CM, Bailey AJ (1979) Cross-linking of collagen in the X-linked Ehlers–Danlos type V. Biochem Biophys Res Comm 88: 281–287

Stewart RE, Hollister DW, Rimoin DL (1977) A new variant of Ehlers–Danlos syndrome: an autosomal dominant disorder of fragile skin, abnormal scarring and generalised periodontitis. Birth Defects 13(3B): 85–93

Sulica VI, Cooper PH, Pope FM, Hambrick GW, Garson BM, McKusick VA (1979) Cutaneous histologic features in Ehlers–Danlos syndrome: study of 21 patients. Arch Dermatol 115(1): 40–42

The illustrations in this chapter appeared in 'The Ehlers–Danlos syndrome' (Beighton 1970) and are reproduced by permission of the publishers, Wm Heinemann Medical Books Ltd.

10. Familial Undifferentiated Hypermobility Syndromes

Introduction

The familial undifferentiated hypermobility syndromes are a heterogeneous group of disorders in which generalised joint laxity is the primary clinical manifestation. The Ehlers–Danlos syndrome (EDS) (Chap. 9) and other rare genetic conditions (Chap. 11) which have additional non-articular stigmata are excluded from this category.

Semantic confusion still occurs, since the term 'hypermobility syndrome' is employed in a clinical context for any patient with articular symptoms which are a consequence of lax joints, in the absence of a specific syndromic diagnosis (see Chap. 5). The major problem lies in distinguishing between individuals who are at the upper end of the spectrum of the normal range of joint movements and those who have an inherited connective tissue disorder which presents with articular laxity (i.e. the familial undifferentiated hyper-mobility syndrome).

The heterogeneity of EDS may lead to problems in diagnosis. The common type I or gravis form of EDS is easily distinguishable by virtue of the dermal extensibility and widespread scarring, but the other types, in which these latter features are less obvious, can cause confusion. Indeed, a sporadic individual with no stigmata other than lax joints may be difficult or impossible to categorise.

It is probable that loose-jointed persons with articular symptoms comprise a very heterogeneous group of simple and complex genetic conditions. The limits of syndromic resolution at a clinical level have been reached and further delineation will depend upon the recognition of specific histological, bio-chemical or molecular markers.

Notwithstanding the problem of syndromic identity, this chapter is con-cerned with the familial undifferentiated hypermobility syndromes as defined in the first paragraph.

Classification of Familial Undifferentiated Hypermobility

Early accounts of familial hypermobility were given by Key (1927) and Sturkie (1941). The generation to generation transmission of loose jointedness in association with multiple dislocations was documented by Hass and Hass (1958) under the designation 'arthrochalasis multiplex congenita'. The patients reported in this article included individuals with EDS and no attempt was made to differentiate the separate entities. (The term 'arthrochalasis multiplex congenita' is now used for EDS VII, with resultant confusion!) Carter and Sweetnam (1958 and 1960) and Carter and Wilkinson (1964) drew further attention to the association of familial generalised joint laxity and dislocations.

In addition to the generalised hypermobility syndromes, familial joint laxity is sometimes localised to a single site. For instance, Whitney (1932) described autosomal dominant inheritance of hypermobility which was confined to the interphalangeal joint of the thumb.

Autosomal Dominant Undifferentiated Generalised Hypermobility

Beighton and Horan (1970) described two families in which joint laxity was transmitted as an autosomal dominant trait. The first was a kindred of contortionists who had experienced few orthopaedic problems during their professional activities, while the second family had multiple dislocations and deformities which were attributable to their hypermobility. It was suggested that these two familial conditions were separate entities and that the variability of complications was indicative of heterogeneity. Case reports and the pedigrees of these families are given below.

Case Reports

Kindred 1. DW, born in 1940, had been a professional contortionist since the age of 17. Her act involved extreme degrees of joint movement, but she did not need to follow a regimen of exercises to retain her mobility. Even after several weeks of inactivity her articular laxity would remain unimpaired. Her general health was good and she had had never experienced orthopaedic disability.

She was an intelligent young woman, 165 cm in height, weighing 51.7 kg. Her stance and gait were normal and she had no musculo-skeletal deformity. She possessed a remarkable degree of articular laxity, achieving the maximum score of 9 out of 9 on the mobility index. Active movements in both shoulder joints included abduction of 240°, flexion of 220° and extension of 90°. The hip joints could be hyperextended 30°, abducted 50°, medially rotated 50° and laterally rotated 110°. The elbow joints could be hyperextended 10° and the knee joints 15°. The wrist and ankle joints were also lax, as were the small joints in the hands and feet. Her abilities are illustrated in Figs. 10.1–10.4

One of her three sisters had marked articular laxity, as had her father. Her paternal grandfather and his brother had been loose-jointed performers in Buffalo Bill's circus. None of these hypermobile individuals had any musculo-skeletal deformity or disability, and significant osteoarthritis did not develop in old age.

Kindred 2. CR was born in 1920 with congenital dislocation of both hips, which were successfully treated by manipulation and plaster casts. She was troubled in infancy by extreme laxity of the ankles and tarsal joints. For this reason she wore surgical boots and arch supports until the age of 12. Recurrent dislocations of both patellae occurred during childhood, and both elbow joints were dislocated in minor falls. When she was 28 years of age she began

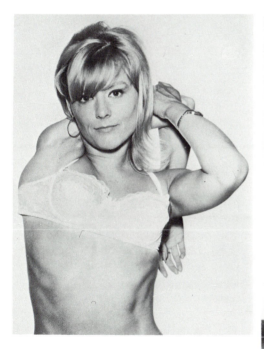

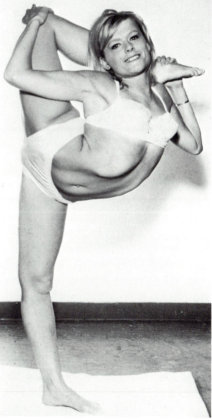

▲
Fig. 10.1. A young woman with familial generalised articular hypermobility. From Beighton (1970).

Fig. 10.2. She was able to maintain her joint ▶ laxity without any special training. From Beighton (1970).

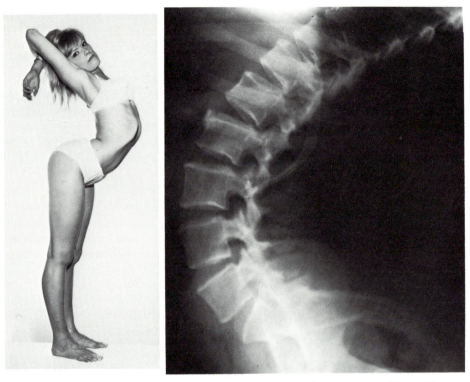

Fig. 10.3. (*left*) Her range of spinal movements was especially impressive. From Beighton (1970).

Fig. 10.4. (*right*) Lateral radiograph of the spine showing the extreme degree of hyperextension that she was able to achieve. From Beighton (1970).

to be troubled by osteoarthritis of the hips. This problem became increasingly severe, and bilateral upper femoral osteotomies were performed when she was 46 years old. She had always been aware of her articular laxity, but the movements of the hips and spine became limited by osteoarthritis during her twenties. At the time of examination, she remarked that it was only the pronounced hyperextensibility of her knees that permitted her to tie her shoe laces. Her general health was good and there had been no serious illness in the past.

At the age of 52 years she was 152 cm in height and weighed 53.5 kg. She had marked thoraco-lumbar kyphoscoliosis and walked with the aid of a stick. Movements of the hips and spine were restricted, but the other joints were very lax. In particular, the metacarpophalangeal joints of the fifth fingers could be extended to 90° and the thumbs could be made to touch either surface of the forearm. Flexion and extension to 90° was possible at the wrist, and the elbows and knees could be hyperextended by 15°. The skin was normal and the other systems were intact.

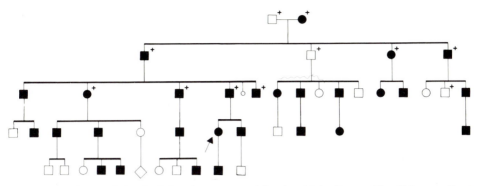

Fig. 10.5. Pedigree of a kindred showing autosomal dominant inheritance of familial generalised articular hypermobility.

Loose-jointedness was present in other members of the kindred, and many of them had orthopaedic problems. These varied in degree and severity: in particular, pes planus and spinal kyphoscoliosis were well-known family traits. The pedigree is shown in Fig. 10.5

The benign hypermobile type III EDS differs from the autosomal dominant familial undifferentiated hypermobility syndrome only by virtue of additional dermal extensibility. If this manifestation is of minor degree, exact diagnostic categorisation may be impossible. This problem is compounded by the fact that an ill-defined velvety texture to the skin and minimal cutaneous extensibility and scarring may be present in both the hypermobility syndrome and type III EDS.

A kindred with joint laxity in four generations and a propensity to recurrent dislocations of the patella was reported by Shapiro et al. (1976). A further family with autosomal dominant generalised joint laxity and multiple disloca-tions was described by Horton el al. (1980). These authors reviewed the literature and proposed the designation 'familial joint instability syndrome' for this entity. They suggested that the term 'familial simple joint laxity' should be employed for the benign familial hypermobility syndrome in which dislocations and orthopaedic complications were unusual.

Autosomal Recessive Undifferentiated Generalised Hypermobility

Autosomal recessive inheritance of undifferentiated hypermobility was recog-nised in two sisters born into a consanguineous French–Canadian kindred (Horan and Beighton 1973). Both had gross generalised joint laxity and a soft velvety skin. The younger sister had experienced numerous orthopaedic problems but the elder was asymptomatic.

Case Report

A French–Canadian girl was born in 1942. For as long as she could remember she had been aware of her unusual degree of joint laxity. She wore corrective shoes for pes planus during childhood. From the age of 12 she had been troubled by instability of her left shoulder joint. Dislocation never occurred, but she could spontaneously sublux the shoulder. She was unable to lift heavy objects with her left arm, and she experienced pain in the shoulder on attempting to carry even a light shopping bag.

When she was 16 years of age, bilateral ankle instability became troublesome, with frequent effusions in both ankles. Bilateral triple arthrodeses were carried out when she was aged 21, and her ankles were subsequently stable and free from pain.

At the age of 20 she began to notice occasional 'clicking' in both hips. This persisted, and it was followed by aching, which passed off with rest. When 23 years old she developed persistent low back pain on standing or sitting for long periods. Intensive physiotherapy and a plaster jacket alleviated the discomfort, but 1 year later she developed radicular pain in the left leg. Myelography showed no evidence of a lumbar disc protrusion. A plaster jacket or brace brought about some improvement, but this pain persisted. Fusion of the L5/S1 disc space was carried out, and during the operation the surgeon noted marked instability at the L4/5 and L5/S1 levels. Thereafter she experienced considerable relief of her symptoms. Apart from her joint problems, her general health was very good.

Examination revealed a pleasant young woman with gross generalised articular hypermobility. Her range of passive joint movements included hyperextension of the metacarpophalangeal joints to 95°, easy apposition of the thumbs to either aspect of the forearm, hyperextension of the elbows to 15° and of the knees to 15°. Her shoulder-girdle joints were extremely lax and the left shoulder joint could be readily subluxated. Her skin was soft and velvety in texture, but not hyperelastic, and there was no evidence of cutaneous fragility. No abnormality was detected in her other systems. Radiographs of the shoulders, hips, and spine did not show any evidence of degenerative joint disease.

The patient's only sibling was an elder sister who also had articular laxity. She could extend her metacarpophalangeal joints to 100°, appose her thumbs to the flexor aspect of her forearm, hyperextend her knees and elbows by 15°, and easily place the palms of her hands on the floor while keeping her legs straight. However, her degree of hypermobility was not as great as her sister's and she had never experienced any orthopaedic problems. Her skin had the same velvety consistency, but examination was otherwise normal.

The sisters' ancestors came from the Angers district in Northern France and settled in Quebec in 1652. There was no doubt that the parents were related, although the precise degree of consanguinity was uncertain (see pedigree, Fig. 10.6). Neither the parents nor any other members of the kindred were known to be hypermobile.

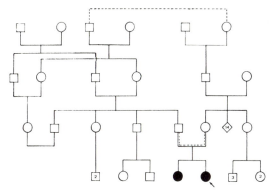

Fig. 10.6. Pedigree of a consanguineous French-Canadian family showing autosomal recessive inheritance of undifferentiated hypermobility.

The autosomal recessive form of the familial undifferentiated hypermobility syndrome is very similar to type VII EDS in which joint laxity is a major feature and the latter differs only by virtue of reduced stature and a characteristic facies. However, the demonstration of a defect on the alpha 2 procollagen peptide in this form of EDS (Steinmann et al. 1979) may permit recognition at a biochemical level.

Articular Complications of Familial Undifferentiated Hypermobility

In some hypermobile families a wide spectrum of dislocations and subluxations may occur, while in others there is a predisposition to dislocation or subluxation of a particular joint (Figs. 10.7 and 10.8). Following the reports of Carter and Sweetnam (1958 and 1960), recurrent dislocation of the patella and shoulder have been repeatedly recorded in families with the hypermobility syndrome. Shapiro et al. (1976) mentioned recurrent patella dislocations in four generations of a loose-jointed kindred.

The occurrence of hip dislocation in families with hypermobility has been documented by Carter and Wilkinson (1964), Wynne-Davis (1970a, b) and Bjerkreim and van der Hagen (1974). Fredensborg (1978) described an unusual patient with unilateral congenital dislocation of the hip and joint laxity which was present only on the same side.

Apart from recurrent dislocations and subluxations, hypermobile individuals are liable to develop other orthopaedic complications due to their joint laxity. These include sprains, effusions, spinal malalignment and pes planus.

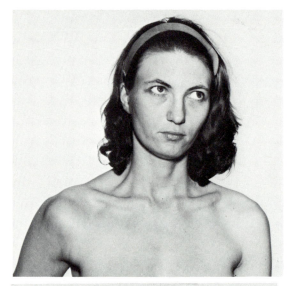

Fig. 10.7. Spontaneous dislocation of the right shoulder in the familial undifferentiated hypermobility syndrome.

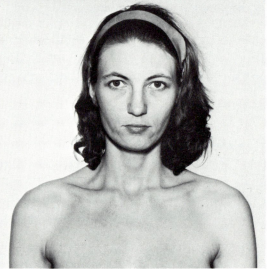

Fig. 10.8. The patient has spontaneously reduced her dislocated shoulder.

Other Phenotypic Manifestations of Familial Undifferentiated Hypermobility

Inguinal herniae are often encountered in hypermobile individuals and it seems likely that they are a genuine complication of the syndrome. In view of the underlying generalised connective tissue abnormality, this tendency to hernia is not unexpected. An association between hypermobility and mitral valve prolapse has recently been recognised (Grahame et al. 1981).

As mentioned in the discussion on differential diagnosis, some persons with the familial undifferentiated hypermobility syndrome have an unusual rubbery or velvety consistency to their skin. This feature is very difficult to quantitate, but nevertheless it is of some value in distinguishing an affected individual from a loose-jointed 'normal' person. In the same way, minor degrees of dermal extensibility and a mild bruising tendency may be present. Again, these are 'soft' stigmata with considerable overlap with normality on one hand, and EDS type III on the other.

References

Beighton P (1970) The Ehlers–Danlos syndrome. William Heinemann Medical Books, London

Beighton P, Horan FT (1970) Dominant inheritance in familial generalised articular hypermobility. J Bone Joint Surg [Br] 52: 145–147

Bjerkreim I, van der Hagen CB (1974) Congenital dislocation of the hip in Norway. Clin Genet 5: 433–448

Carter C, Sweetnam R (1958) Familial joint laxity and recurrent dislocations of the patella. J Bone Joint Surg [Br] 40: 664–667

Carter C, Sweetnam R (1960) Recurrent dislocation of the patella and of the shoulder, their association with familial joint laxity. J Bone Joint Surg [Br] 42: 721–727

Carter C, Wilkinson J (1964) Persistent joint laxity and congenital dislocation of the hip. J Bone Joint Surg [Br] 46: 40–45

Fredensborg N (1978) Unilateral joint laxity in unilateral congenital dislocation of the hip. Orthop 2/2: 177–178

Grahame R, Edwards JC, Pitcher D, Gabell A, Harvey W (1981) A clinical and echocardiographic study of patients with the hypermobility syndrome. Ann Rheum Dis 40: 541–546

Hass J, Hass R (1958), Arthrochalasis multiplex congenita. J Bone Joint Surg [Am] 40: 663–674

Horan FT, Beighton P (1973) Recessive inheritance of generalized joint hypermobility. Rheum Rehab 12: 47–49

Horton WA, Collins DL, DeSmet AA, Kennedy JA, Schimke RN (1980) Familial joint instability syndrome. Am J Med Genet 6: 221–228

Key JA (1927) Hypermobility of joints as a sex-linked hereditary characteristic. JAMA 88: 1710–1712

Shapiro SD, Jorgenson RJ, Salinas CF (1976) Recurrent dislocation of the patella versus generalized joint laxity. The National Foundation. Birth Defects. XII (5): 287–291

Steinmann B, Tuderman L, Martin GR, Prockop DJ (1979) Evidence for a structural mutation of procollagen in a patient with Ehlers–Danlos syndrome type VII. Eur J Pediat 130: 203–205

Sturkie PD (1941) Hypermobile joints in all descendants for two generations. J Hered 32: 232–234

Whitney LF (1932) Inheritance of double-jointedness of the thumb. J Hered 23: 425–426

Wynne-Davis R (1970) Acetabular dysplasia and familial joint laxity, two etiologic factors in congenital dislocation of the hip. J Bone Joint Surg [Br] 52: 704–716

Wynne-Davis R (1970) A familial study of neonatal and late-diagnosis congenital dislocation of the hip. J Med Genet 7: 315–333

11. Miscellaneous Joint Laxity Syndromes

In addition to the Ehlers–Danlos syndrome (EDS) (Chap. 9) and the familial undifferentiated hypermobility syndromes (Chap. 10), joint laxity is present in a number of inherited disorders. In some it is a major feature, while in others the hypermobility is overshadowed by other syndromic components.

Joint Laxity in Inherited Connective Tissue Disorders

Hypermobility is a clinically important facet of a few well-established connective tissue disorders, the most important of which are the Marfan syndrome and osteogenesis imperfecta. A full description of these conditions and related disorders can be found in 'Heritable Disorders of Connective Tissue' (McKusick 1972).

Marfan Syndrome

The hallmarks of the Marfan syndrome are disproportionate limb length in relation to the trunk and arachnodactyly (long slim digits). Thoracic asymmetry and spinal malalignment are sometimes present and dislocation of the ocular lenses and aortic and mitral valvular disease are additional features (Fig. 11.1). Aneurysmal dissection of the aorta in adulthood is a common mode of death.

Joint laxity is maximal in the wrists, but other joints may be hypermobile to some degree (Figs. 11.2 and 11.3). Orthopaedic complications which are related to the laxity include recurrent dislocation, especially of the shoulder and patella, spinal malalignment, pes planus and hallux valgus.

Inheritance is autosomal dominant but phenotypic expression is very variable and mildly affected persons may be difficult to distinguish from normal individuals.

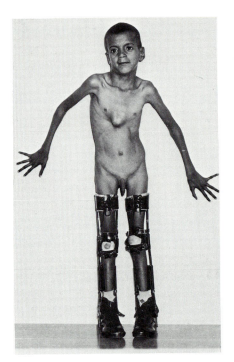

Fig. 11.1. A boy with the Marfan syndrome; arachnodactyly and thoracic asymmetry are evident.

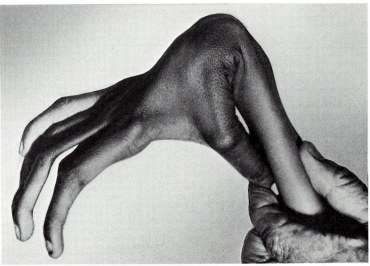

Fig. 11.2. Articular laxity is maximal in the wrist joint in the Marfan syndrome.

Marfanoid Hypermobility Syndrome

The Marfanoid hypermobility syndrome is a rare autosomal recessive disorder in which a marfanoid habitus is associated with gross generalised

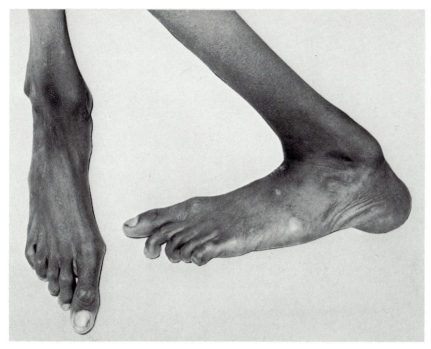

Fig. 11.3. The feet are excessively long and the ankles are lax in this patient with the Marfan syndrome.

articular hypermobility and marked dermal extensibility (Walker et al. 1969). Ocular complications do not occur but coarctation of the aorta has been recorded (Daneshwar et al. 1979). A number of reported patients have been regarded as having a combination of EDS and the classic Marfan syndrome (Birkenstock et al. 1973), but it is probable that the marfanoid hypermobility syndrome represents a distinct syndromic entity. Spinal malalignment, genu recurvatum and recurrent dislocations may result from the joint laxity.

Osteogenesis Imperfecta

Osteogenesis imperfecta (OI) is a common and well-known disorder in which bone fragility is associated with blue sclerae and wormian bones in the skull (Figs. 11.4 and 11.5).

Hypermobility of the digits is obvious in some affected persons and in a minority joint laxity may be widespread. In a review of the historical background of OI, Weil (1981) drew attention to several reports in the early literature of hypermobility and recurrent dislocations. Ligamentous laxity probably plays a significant role in the development of the spinal deformities which occur in a proportion of individuals with OI (Benson and Newman 1981).

Osteogenesis imperfecta is undoubtedly heterogeneous and the presence or absence of articular laxity may serve as a diagnostic discriminant.

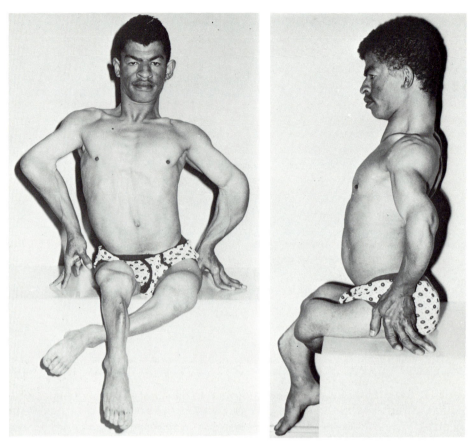

Fig. 11.4. (*left*) A young man with osteogenesis imperfecta, showing severe deformity of the long bones and spine.

Fig. 11.5. (*right*) The digits are sometimes lax in osteogenesis imperfecta, as in this patient.

Other Bone Fragility–Joint Laxity Syndromes

In the osteoporosis—pseudoglioma syndrome the radiological appearance of the skeleton and the presence of wormian bones are reminiscent of OI. These features are associated with mild mental retardation and blindness in infancy due to pseudogliomatous retinal detachment and other ocular complications (Bianchine and Murdoch 1972; Neuhauser et al. 1976). Ligamentous laxity is present, but does not cause clinical problems. Approximately ten patients have been reported and inheritance is autosomal recessive.

Using the designation 'OI associated with the Ehlers–Danlos syndrome' Biering and Iverson (1955) reported the occurrence of gross generalised osteoporosis, fractures, articular laxity with dislocations, dermal extensibility and blue sclerae. Subsequently, Meigel et al. (1974) described an autosomal recessive syndrome of bone fragility and marked joint laxity in a single individual. The sclerae and skin were normal in this patient.

A family with autosomal recessive inheritance of blue sclerae, keratoconus, deafness and spondylolisthesis was described by Greenfield et al. (1973). Biglan et al. (1977) reported five patients from two families with a similar disorder in which keratoglobus, blue sclerae, hearing loss, mottling of the teeth and generalised joint laxity were the main features. Inheritance was autosomal recessive. Robertson (1975) detected hypermobility in 50% of a series of 44 patients with keratoconus, and made a reasonable suggestion that the ocular and ligamentous abnormalities shared a common pathogenesis.

Larsen Syndrome

The Larsen syndrome is characterised by marked generalised hypermobility in association with stunted stature, mid-facial hypoplasia, flattening of the nasal bridge and spatulate digits (Figs. 11.6 and 11.7: Larsen et al. 1950; Latta et al. 1971; Harris and Cullen 1971; Robertson et al. 1975). Joint laxity is maximal in the knees and genu recurvatum and instability commonly occur.

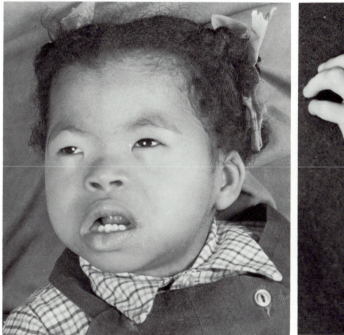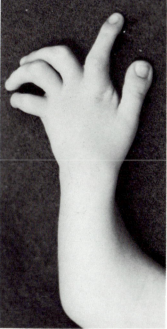

Fig. 11.6. (*left*) A girl with the Larsen syndrome showing epicanthus and the characteristic broad flat nasal bridge.

Fig. 11.7. (*right*) In the Larsen syndrome the digits are lax and their tips are spatulate.

Initial presentation is as a 'floppy infant' and other complications include dislocation of the hips and radial heads, and talipes equinovarus. In later childhood the ligamentous laxity predisposes to spinal malalignment, which may be progressive and difficult to manage.

It is likely that there are distinct mild autosomal dominant and severe autosomal recessive forms of the syndrome.

Joint Laxity in Dwarfism

Generalised or localised hypermobility is a component of several inherited skeletal dysplasias in which dwarfism is the major feature.

Spondylo-epi-metaphyseal Dysplasia with Joint Laxity and Severe Progressive Kyphoscoliosis

A series of seven children with skeletal dysplasia, gross generalised joint laxity and severe spinal malalignment were reported by Beighton and Kozlowski (1980: Fig. 11.8). The skin was rubbery and extensible but not fragile (Fig. 11.9). Numerous orthopaedic problems were related to the hypermobility, including dislocation, subluxation, genu valgum, genu recurvatum, talipes equinovarus and pes planus. Inheritance is probably autosomal recessive.

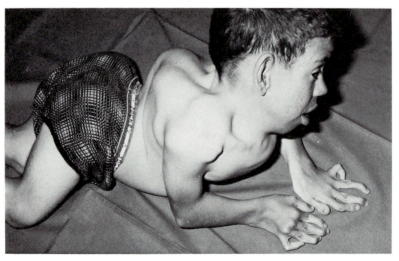

Fig. 11.8. A boy with a form of spondylo-epi-metaphyseal dysplasia (SEMD) in which gross kyphoscoliosis and articular laxity are major features.

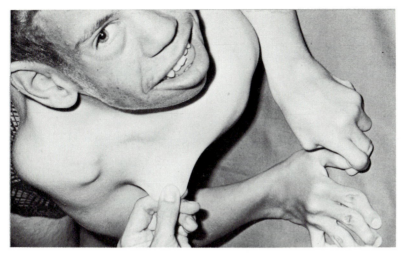

Fig. 11.9. The skin is extensible but not fragile in this form of SEMD.

Pseudoachondroplasia

Pseudoachondroplasia is a comparatively common dwarfing skeletal dysplasia in which joint laxity is a variable component (Fig. 11.10). The digits are
often stubby with an impressive range of movement. In some persons the
hypermobility is sufficiently severe to cause dislocations, deformities and
spinal malalignment, while in others articular movements are normal. It is
probable that these variable stigmata are indicative of heterogeneity. There is
good evidence in favour of autosomal dominant and autosomal recessive
forms of pseudoachondroplasia (Hall 1975; Kozlowski 1976; Heselson et al.
1977) but at present delineation is incomplete.

Morquio Syndrome (MPS IV)

The eponymous designation 'Morquio' is sometimes applied to any dwarfing
syndrome in which spinal malalignment is a major feature, but in the strict
sense the term pertains to mucopolysaccharidosis type IV (MPS IV).
Dwarfism, thoracic deformity, aortic incompetence and progressive corneal
clouding are the major clinical features, and the diagnosis may be confirmed
by demonstration of the radiographic changes of dysostosis multiplex and
excessive excretion of keratosulphate in the urine.

In distinction to the other mucopolysaccharidoses the joints are lax. This is
most obvious in the digits, but the hypermobility also predisposes to
orthopaedic complications including genu valgum, spinal malalignment and
pes planus (Fig. 11.11). It is of special clinical importance that the odontoid

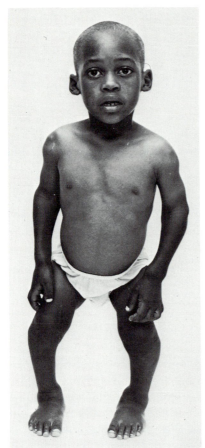

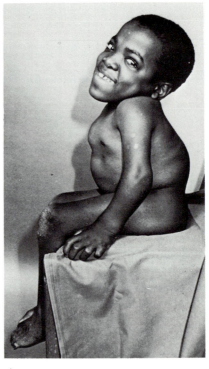

Fig. 11.11. A boy with MPS IV showing the typical barrel chest, short neck and spinal malalignment. The digital laxity which is present in this condition is a useful diagnostic discriminant from the other mucopolysaccharidoses.

Fig. 11.10. Pseudoachondroplasia; short limbed dwarfism and genu varum are the major stigmata. Loose stubby digits are characteristic of some forms of this heretogeneous disorder.

process is often hypoplastic in MPS IV, as the combination of this defect and joint laxity places affected persons at risk of subluxation of the cervical spine and cord compression (Greenberg 1968; Beighton and Craig 1973).

Other Dwarfing Dysplasias

Cartilage-hair hypoplasia or metaphyseal chondrodysplasia type McKusick is characterised by fine hair, disproportionate dwarfism and lax stubby digits. There is a propensity to Hirschsprung disease and severe varicella. The condition has been extensively studied among inbred Amish community of Pennsylvania (McKusick et al. 1965; Lowry et al. 1970).

Hypochondroplasia is a relatively common dwarfing dysplasia in which the clinical and radiographic features are similar to but milder than those of achondroplasia. There may be some generalised joint laxity, but this rarely causes clinical problems (Beals 1969).

The digits are hypermobile in acromesomelic dysplasia (Beighton 1974) and the knee joints are lax in the Ellis van Creveld syndrome (McKusick et al. 1964). Hypermobility is also present in the classical form of spondylo-epiphyseal dysplasia congenita (Spranger and Langer 1970). These disorders are all rare, and unlikely to be encountered in routine practice.

Rare Genetic Syndromes in Which Hypermobility Is Overshadowed by Other Manifestations

Hajdu–Cheney syndrome

The Hajdu–Cheney syndrome is a rare autosomal dominant disorder which was first identified in a small family in Michigan, USA. The major stigmata are acro-osteolysis, osteoporosis, hypoplasia of the mandible, stunted stature, bone fragility, early loss of teeth and multiple wormian bones (Brown et al. 1976; Weleber and Beals 1976). Articular laxity is a variable feature which does not cause significant complications.

Hyperlysinaemia

Hyperlysinaemia is an autosomal recessive and possibly heterogeneous condition in which marked generalised joint laxity is associated with mental retardation and convulsions (Ghadimi et al. 1965). The ligamentous laxity plays an important role in the initial presentation as a 'floppy infant' and may be related to the subluxation of the ocular lenses which occurs in some affected persons (Smith et al. 1971).

FG Syndrome (Opitz–Kaveggia)

The Opitz–Kaveggia FG syndrome is an X-linked multiple malformation disorder in which a characteristic facies, mental retardation and imperforate anus are the most consistent features. The designation 'FG' is derived from the initials of the patients' surnames, and about 15 affected boys have been reported (Opitz and Kaveggia 1974; Riccardi et al. 1977). Articular laxity predisposes to sloping shoulders, lumbar lordosis and club feet.

C Syndrome (Opitz Trigonocephaly Syndrome)

The C syndrome is a very rare multiple malformation complex and the seven reported patients have all died in infancy. The major features are very short limbs, an abnormal facies and redundant skin (Opitz et al. 1969; Oberklaid and Danks 1975). The joints are very extensible, especially the knees, and in one patient autopsy revealed poorly developed ligaments at the knee joint. Inheritance is presumably autosomal recessive.

Tricho-rhino-phalangeal Syndrome, Type II (Langer-Giedion Syndrome)

The manifestations of the tricho-rhino-phalangeal syndrome (TRP) type II, of which seven cases have been reported, resemble those of the better-known TRP type I. The most obvious features are sparse scalp hair, a bulbous nose and cone-shaped phalangeal epiphyses. Mental retardation and multiple exostoses are discriminant features in TRP type II (Hall et al. 1975; Kozlowski et al. 1977). Articular laxity is variable, but may cause spinal curvature and lead to presentation as a 'floppy infant'. The genetic basis is unknown.

X-Linked Cutis Laxa

Autosomal dominant and recessive forms of cutis laxa are well-established and an X-linked variety has now been delineated. These latter patients have cutaneous laxity and the additional features of scar formation, thoracic deformity and mild generalised joint laxity. Lysyl oxidase activity is deficient (Byers et al. 1976).

The condition of bone dystrophy, articular hypermobility and dermal laxity studied by Debré et al. (1937) in French siblings is a similar entity. As a female was affected in this kindred, the disorder could not be X-linked and autosomal recessive inheritance is likely.

Aarskog Syndrome

The main features of the Aarskog syndrome are short stature, a shawl scrotum and a characteristic facies (Aarskog 1970). The metacarpophalangeal joints are very lax and when they are extended concomitant flexion occurs at the proximal interphalangeal joints. The hypermobility is sometimes generalised with secondary consequences such as genu recurvatum, pes planus and metatarsus adductus. Hypermobility of the cervical spine in conjunction with odontoid hypoplasia may lead to spinal cord compression. Inheritance is probably X-linked recessive, although sex-influenced autosomal dominant inheritance has been postulated (Sugarman et al. 1973).

Cohen Syndrome

The major features of the Cohen syndrome are variable mental retardation, truncal obesity with onset in the first decade, muscle hypotonia, narrow hands and feet and delayed puberty. Generalised joint laxity predisposes to genu valgum and spinal malalignment (Carey and Bryan 1978; Balestrazzi et al. 1980).

Night Blindness, Characteristic Facies and Hyperextensibility

Hunter et al. (1979) described two Canadian brothers with an unusual facies, slowly progressive night blindness, myopia and generalised joint laxity. The mode of inheritance was uncertain.

Multiple Endocrine Neoplasia Type III

Persons with a multiple endocrine neoplasia syndrome type III have a Marfanoid habitus, a characteristic facies and a propensity to medullary thyroid carcinoma and phaeochromocytoma. Abdominal symptoms may result from colonic ganglioneuromata. Joint laxity leads to spinal malalignment, genu valgum and foot deformity (Schimke et al. 1968; Gorlin and Mirkin 1972). Inheritance is autosomal dominant.

Coffin-Siris Syndrome

The syndrome described by Coffin and Siris (1970) comprises microcephaly, mental retardation, growth impairment, sparse hair, hypoplasia of the nails of the fifth fingers and a coarse facies. Lucaya et al. (1981) reported 4 cases, reviewed 12 others from the literature, and drew attention to the presence of joint laxity in affected persons. The genetic background is uncertain.

Peculiar Face, Pectus Carinatum and Joint Laxity

A Mexican brother and sister with an unusual facies, thoracic deformity and generalised joint laxity were reported by Guizar-Vazquez et al. (1980). The additional features of pes planus and genu valgum were probably the result of the hypermobility. Autosomal recessive inheritance was postulated.

References

Aarskog D (1970) A familial syndrome of short stature associated with facial dysplasia and genital anomalies. J Pediatr 77: 856–861

Balestrazzi P, Corrini L, Villani G, Bolla MP, Càsa F, Bernasconi S (1980) The Cohen syndrome: clinical and endocrinological studies of two new cases. J Med Genet 17: 430–432

Beals RK (1969) Hypochondroplasia. J Bone Joint Surg [Am] 51: 728–739

Beighton P, Craig J (1973) Atlanto-axial dislocation in the Morquio syndrome. J Bone Joint Surg [Br] 55: 478–480

Beighton P (1974) Autosomal recessive inheritance in the mesomelic dwarfism of Campailla and Martinelli. Clin Genet 5: 363–367

Beighton PH, Kozlowski K (1980) Spondylo-epi-metaphyseal dysplasia with joint laxity and severe progressive kyphoscoliosis. Skeletal Radiol 5: 205–212

Benson DR, Newman DC (1981) The spine and surgical treatment in osteogenesis imperfecta. Clin Orthop 159: 147–153

Bianchine JW, Murdoch JL (1969) Juvenile osteoporosis (?) in a boy with bilateral enucleation of the eyes for pseudoglioma. The clinical delineation of birth defects. IV. Skeletal dysplasias. Birth Defects V (4): 225–226

Biering A, Iverson T (1955) Osteogenesis imperfecta associated with Ehlers–Danlos syndrome. Acta Paediatr Scand 44: 279–283

Biglan AW, Brown SI, Johnson BL (1977) Keratoglobus and blue sclerae. Am J Ophthalmol 83/2: 225–233

Birkenstock WE, Louw JH, Maze A, Sladen RN (1973) Combined Ehlers–Danlos and Marfan's syndromes with a case report. SA Med J 47: 2097–2102

Brown DM, Bradford DS, Gorlin RJ, Desnick RJ, Langer LO Jr, Jowsey J, Sauk JJ Jr (1976) The acro-osteolysis syndrome: morphologic and biochemical studies. J Pediatr 88: 573–580

Byers, PH, Narayanan AS, Bornstein P, Hall JG (1976) An X-linked form of cutis laxa due to deficiency of lysyloxidase. Birth Defects 12(No 5): 293–298

Carey JC, Bryan DH (1978) Confirmation of the Cohen syndrome. J Pediatr 93: 239–244

Coffins GS, Siris E (1970) Mental retardation with absent fifth fingernail and terminal phalanx. Am J Dis Child 119: 433–439

Daneshwar A, Tavakol D, Nozarian J (1979) Marfanoid hypermobility syndrome associated with coarctation of the aorta. Br Heart J 41(5): 621–623

Debré R, Marie J, Seringe P (1937) 'Cutis laxa' avec dystrophies osseuses. Bull Mem Soc Med Hosp Paris 53: 1038–1039

Ghadimi H, Binnington VI, Pecora P (1965) Hyperlysinemia associated with mental retardation. New Eng J Med 273: 723–729

Gorlin RJ, Mirkin BL (1972) Multiple mucosal neuromas, phaeochromocytama, medullary carcinoma of the thyroid and marfanoid body build with muscle wasting. Syndrome of hyperplasia and neoplasia of neural crest derivatives. A unitarian concept. Z Kinderheilk 113: 313–321

Greenberg AD (1968) Atlantoaxial dislocation. Brain 91: 655–684

Greenfield G, Romano A, Stein R, Goodman RM (1973) Blue sclerae and keratoconus: Key features of a district heritable disorder of connective tissue. Clin Genet 4: 8–16

Guizar–Vazquez J, Sanchez G, Manzano C (1980) Peculiar face, pectus carinatum and joint laxity in brother and sister. Clin Genet 18/4: 280–283

Hall BD, Langer LO, Giedion A, Smith DW, Cohen MM, Beals RK, Bradner M (1974) Langer–Giedion syndrome. Birth Defects ×(12): 147–164

Hall JG (1975) Pseudoachondroplasia. Birth Defects XI(6): 187–202

Harris R, Cullen CH (1971) Autosomal dominant inheritance in Larsen's syndrome. Clin Genet 2: 87–90

Heselson NG, Cremin BJ, Beighton P (1977) Pseudoachondroplasia, a report of 13 cases. Br J Radiol 50: 473–482

Hunter AGW, Thompson DR, Reed MH, Macrodimitris AG (1979) Night blindness, characteristic facies, and skeletal abnormalities in two brothers. J Med Genet 16/4: 309–313

Kozlowski K (1976) Pseudoachondroplastic dysplasia (Maroteaux–Lamy). Austral Radiol 20: 255–269

Kozlowski K, Harrington G, Barylak A, Bartoszewica B (1977) Multiple exostoses–mental retardation syndrome (Ale-Calo or M.E.M.R. syndrome): description of two childhood cases. Clin Pediatr 11: 219–224

Larsen LJ, Schottstaedt ER, Bost FC (1950) Multiple congenital dislocations associated with characteristic facial abnormality. J Pediatr 37: 574–581

Latta RJ, Graham CB, Aase J, Scham SM, Smith DW (1971) Larsen's syndrome: a skeletal dysplasia with multiple joint dislocations and unusual facies. J Pediatr 78: 291–298

Lucaya J, Garcia-Conesa JA, Bosch-Banyeras JM, Pons–Peradejordi G (1981) The Coffin–Siris syndrome. A report of four cases and review of the literature. Pediatr Radiol 11(1): 35–38

Lowry RB, Wood BJ, Birkbeck JA, Padwick PH (1970) Cartilage–hair hypoplasia. A rare and recessive cause of dwarfism. Clin Pediatr 9: 44–46

McKusick VA, Egeland JA, Eldridge R, Krusen DE (1964) Dwarfism in the Amish. The Ellis-van Creveld syndrome. Bull Johns Hopkins Hosp 115: 306

McKusick VA, Eldridge R, Hostetler JA, Egeland JA, Ruangwit U (1965) Dwarfism in the Amish. II. Cartilage-hair hypoplasia. Bull Johns Hopkins Hosp 116: 285–326

McKusick VA (1972) Heritable disorders of connective tissue, 4th edn. CV Mosby Co, St Louis

Meigel WN, Muller PK, Pontz BF, Sorrensen N, Spranger J (1974) A constitutional disorder of connective tissue suggesting a defect in collagen synthesis. Klin Wochenschr 52: 906–910

Neuhauser G, Kaveggia EG, Opitz JM (1976) Autosomal recessive syndrome of pseudoglioma-tous blindness, osteoporosis and mild mental retardation. Clin Genet 9: 324–332

Oberklaid F, Danks DM (1975) The Opitz trigonocephaly syndrome: a case report. Am J Dis Child 129: 1348–1349

Opitz JM, Johnson RC, McCreadie SR, Smith DW (1969) The C syndrome of multiple congenital anomalies. The clinical delineation of birth defects. II. Malformation syndromes. Birth Defects. V(2): 161–166

Opitz JM, Kaveggia EG (1974) The FG syndrome. An X-linked recessive syndrome of multiple congenital anomalies and mental retardation. Z Kinderheilk 117: 1–18

Riccardi VM, Hassler E, Lubinsky MS (1977) The FG syndrome: further characterization, report of a third family, and of a sporadic case. Am J Med Genet 1: 47–58

Robertson FW (1975) Keratoconus and the Ehlers–Danlos syndrome; a new aspect of keratoco-nus. Med J Aust 1(18): 571–573

Robertson FW, Kozlowski K, Middleton RW (1975) Larsen's syndrome. Three cases with multiple congenital joint dislocations and distinctive facies. Clin Genet 14: 53–60

Schimke RN, Hartmann WH, Prout TE, Rimoin DL (1968) Phaeochromocytoma, medullary thyroid carcinoma and multiple neuromas. New Eng J Med 279: 1–7

Smith TH, Holland MG, Woody NC (1971) Ocular manifestations of familial hyperlysinemia? Trans Am Acad Ophthalmol Otolaryngol 75: 355–360

Spranger J, Langer LO (1970) Spondyloepiphyseal dysplasia congenita. Radiol 94: 313–322

Sugarman GI, Rimoin DL, Lachman RS (1973) The facial-digital-genital (Aarskog) syndrome. Am J Dis Child 126: 248–252

Walker BA, Beighton PH, Murdoch JL (1969) The Marfanoid hypermobility syndrome. Ann Int Med 71: 349–352

Weil UH (1981) Osteogenesis imperfecta. Clin Orthop 159: 6–10

Weleber RG, Beals RK (1976) Hadju–Cheney syndrome—report of 2 cases and review of literature. J Pediatr 88: 243–249

Subject Index